ACTIVISM
AGAINST AIDS

ACTIVISM AGAINST AIDS

At the Intersections of Sexuality, Race, Gender, and Class

Brett C. Stockdill

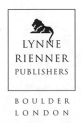

LYNNE
RIENNER
PUBLISHERS

BOULDER
LONDON

Published in the United States of America in 2003 by
Lynne Rienner Publishers, Inc.
1800 30th Street, Boulder, Colorado 80301
www.rienner.com

and in the United Kingdom by
Lynne Rienner Publishers, Inc.
3 Henrietta Street, Covent Garden, London WC2E 8LU

Library of Congress Cataloging-in-Publication Data
Stockdill, Brett C., 1966–
   Activism against AIDS : at the intersections of sexuality, race, gender,
and class / Brett C. Stockdill.
      p. cm.
   Includes bibliographical references and index.
   Contents: AIDS, multiple inequalities, and activism—Framing the AIDS
   crisis: inequalities and divisions on the movement and community levels—
   Forging unity: grassroots AIDS activism in communities of color—ACTing UP
   for prisoners with AIDS: AIDS activism on multiple fronts—Cops, courts, and
   the FBI: repression and AIDS activism—An intersectional approach to social
   movement research and activism.
ISBN 1-58826-111-5 (hbk. : alk. paper)
   1. AIDS (Disease)—Social aspects. 2. AIDS activists. I. Title.
RA643.8 .S765   2003
362.1'969792—dc21   2002073969

British Cataloguing in Publication Data
A Cataloguing in Publication record for this book
is available from the British Library.

Printed and bound in the United States of America

       The paper used in this publication meets the requirements
   ∞ of the American National Standard for Permanence of
       Paper for Printed Library Materials Z39.48-1984.

   5 4 3 2 1

To my parents, Joyce and James Stockdill,
who taught me to work for justice

In memory of all those who have died of AIDS

Contents

Preface

As I developed my proposal for this research project nearly a decade ago, I sought a way to challenge the contention that I could not be both an activist and a sociologist. At Northwestern University, I faced constant pressure to be one or the other. Whereas initial drafts leaned toward the academic side of the fence, I have tried to make this book more accessible to nonsociologists. At the same time, I hope it presents an analysis useful to sociologists and other academics studying social movements.

My research grew out of a sense of urgency regarding the AIDS crisis. As a graduate student in the early 1990s, I found myself looking week after week at the obituaries in the *Windy City Times* and other gay and lesbian newspapers in Chicago and around the country and seeing far too many of my gay brothers and sisters dying of AIDS. At the same time, other oppressed groups, including injection drug users, poor people, and people of color, were dying of AIDS, and their deaths often went unacknowledged. These often overlapping communities witnessed genocidal neglect amid massive death throughout the 1980s, the first decade of the AIDS crisis. It was within this context that I began this book.

I joined ACT UP/Chicago (AIDS Coalition to Unleash Power, Chicago) in the fall of 1992, and on December 1, 1992—World AIDS Day—I eagerly participated in a sit-in at the State of Illinois Build-

ing to protest the state's inadequate response to the AIDS crisis. So
began my research for the book, as well as the next chapter of my
own activism, which until that point had been concentrated in antiracist struggles. As sociologists, we are typically taught to be "objective" when researching social phenomena—as if one could (or
should) be neutral on such issues as AIDS, rape, poverty, police brutality, or environmental injustice. To attempt to be "objective," to *not*
get involved, always seemed to me not only unconscionable in a
moral sense but also less intellectually fulfilling. In ACT
UP/Chicago, especially in the Prison Issues Committee, I found not
only wonderfully compassionate and courageous comrades, but people whose political analyses came from their experiences as activists
more so than from any academic degrees they might have. I learned
a great deal from them and from the prisoners we worked with, people who, in contrast to common stereotypes, were caring and
thoughtful as they lived with and struggled against HIV/AIDS behind
the prison walls. Such involvement provided insight that would have
been inaccessible to a bystander pretending to be objective.

The research phase took about two years. After conducting interviews with AIDS activists in Los Angeles, Chicago, and New York,
I continued my work with ACT UP/Chicago and began writing. It
was during this time that I was infected and diagnosed with HIV myself. Amid the drama of betrayal, self-blame, depression, and fear, I
recognized on a gut level that we had been doing the right thing by
"ACTing UP" in the streets, by being out and queer, and by challenging the criminal justice system and other oppressive institutions
and systems that fuel the AIDS crisis. With the support of family,
friends, and comrades, I completed my doctorate in 1996.

During the years since I finished graduate school, I have constantly been reminded of the growing immensity of the AIDS crisis—
as I deal with my own experiences living as an "out" gay man with
HIV, as I worked at the Services for HIV Prevention, Education,
Care, Treatment, and Reserch for Underserved Minorities (SPEC-
TRUM) mental health clinic in South Central Los Angeles, and as I
learned about the continued catastrophic effect of AIDS throughout
the world, particularly in Africa. I also came to realize that in more
than one way, I owe my life to AIDS activism, in particular to those
who struggled before I joined ACT UP, many of whom died fighting
the AIDS crisis. From this vantage point, I offer this book to readers
as sociological research on a small but significant part of AIDS activism in the United States.

The AIDS crisis is a complex and tragic international social problem. In turn, individual and collective responses to HIV/AIDS have been widespread and have varied greatly. This book is in no way a comprehensive treatment of the AIDS crisis and AIDS activism. What I have attempted to do is describe and analyze several collective efforts targeting AIDS in Los Angeles, Chicago, and New York. These efforts provide insight into challenging AIDS in multiply marginalized populations such as gay and bisexual men of color and prisoners. Such examples are particularly relevant, given the decimation caused by HIV/AIDS in these and other oppressed communities in the United States, as well as in less industrialized nations, particularly the third world. My hope is that this analysis will contribute to current efforts to understand and combat the epidemic.

I also hope that my book will encourage students and scholars of social movements, as well as activists, to think critically about how *multiple* oppressions impact activism. Still today, there are academics and activists who insist on looking at or responding to one form of inequality in isolation—as if that particular inequality were the only one that exists. In other cases, some have prioritized the fight against one "ism" above others. My activism and my research indicate that such an approach inevitably ignores entire segments of communities affected by AIDS and promotes alienation and conflict within these communities. For example, mainstream AIDS activism has often failed to consider the deadly impact of HIV/AIDS on prisoners—reflecting a failure to think critically about race, class, and incarceration within the context of AIDS. Here, I am not arguing that every social-movement organization should try to tackle every issue and cause or attempt to mobilize every community. I am not advocating a "laundry list" approach. Activist organizations (and research projects) should have focus. However, we must be aware of the complex web of issues and inequities that connect each "focus." We must be attentive to what "else" is going on outside our particular areas of action because communities intersect and issues interlock. If we dig a bit deeper, we see that seemingly separate social problems are rooted in the same apparatus of injustice and exploitation. For activists, coalition building is crucial to this effort. Coalitions that promote inclusivity and mindfulness of the interconnectedness of different oppressions are essential. As a whole, the interviews for this book, as well as my participant observation in ACT UP, demonstrate that collective struggles against all forms of oppression are essential in eradicating the AIDS crisis and ultimately creating a more just and humane world.

Acknowledgments

Throughout the various stages of this project, I have received extremely valuable insight and support from a number of people. I would like to thank the prisoners in Illinois and other states who provided vital information to ACT UP/Chicago that is included in this book. Their perseverance and compassion have been remarkable. Former prisoner Virgil Thompson's efforts to work from the "inside" to educate other prisoners about HIV/AIDS and to advocate for more effective AIDS programs and services were especially inspiring and informative.

I would like to thank all the interview respondents who took time from their busy schedules to tell me about their experiences in the trenches of AIDS activism, their ideas about political organizing, and their visions of social change. These interviews were made possible in large part by activists who helped to set up interviews and made critical suggestions for my research, including David Maurrasse and Suzanne Shende in New York City and Emery Smith in Los Angeles.

The members of ACT UP/Chicago enriched my research with discussions on various aspects of AIDS activism. In particular, I would like to thank the members of the Prison Issues Committee, who provided political sustenance during an important period of my life: Jeff Edwards, Kim Feicke, Joyce Fitzgerald, Debbie Gould, Jeanne Kracher, and Betty Pejko.

I would like to thank Aldon Morris, Bernie Beck, and Tom Cook at Northwestern University. Their constructive criticism and guidance were key throughout the different stages of my research and writing.

I would not have been able to come this far without the solidarity of other sociologists who have chosen to defy convention and make a difference as both scholars and activists. During graduate school, my friendships with David Maurrasse, Lisa Park, David Pellow, and Michelle Vannatta helped me in countless ways. Their encouragement on political, academic, and personal levels has kept me going during the tough times. Thanks especially to Lisa and David P. for their thorough reading of the book manuscript. I would also like to thank Saa Meroe, whose brilliant intellect, righteous anger, and sharp wit helped me to maintain focus on the human side of academic research during my postdoctoral fellowship at the University of California at Los Angeles.

Throughout the years, I have derived much inspiration from my students, including Julia Rhoads at Northwestern University and Tyia Wilson at UCLA, as well as Vida Hernandez, Esther Portillo, and Rosa Serna at California State Polytechnic University at Pomona. Thank you to Corissa Hernandez for her careful proofreading of the book. I would like to extend a special thank you to my friend and former student assistant at Cal Poly Pomona, Sergio Antoniuk, who made critical contributions in the areas of research and editing and provided much-needed moral support during times of stress.

There are several other key people I would like to thank at Cal Poly Pomona. As the Behavioral Sciences Department chair, Gary Cretser offered support and took time out of his sabbatical to carefully read the book manuscript and offer helpful comments. Jim Sturges also provided very constructive suggestions on the book draft. College of Letters, Arts, and Social Sciences dean Barbara Way provided much-needed release time during the final stages of the book. My friend Jonnie Owens has served as a wonderful source of queer camaraderie. Finally, my relationship with Mary Yu Danico— as friend, colleague, and family—has been a vital (and fun) part of my physical, emotional, and professional survival and achievements over the past four years.

I give special thanks to Debbie Gould, who has served not only as an ACT UP comrade and friend but also as one of the external reviewers for this book. Her comprehensive review helped me to strengthen the book analytically and substantively.

I would like to thank Bridget Julian at Lynne Rienner Publishers for her belief in this project and her support, which have been crucial in the completion of the book. In addition, I would like to thank the other members of Lynne Rienner Publishers, including Lesli Athanasoulis, Beth Partin, and Liz Miles for their important contributions to the book.

While in Chicago and Los Angeles (and a few other places, too!), I have been lucky to have some wonderful friends who have listened to me complain, given me support, and made me laugh. *Muchas gracias* to Crissy Booker, Linda Evans, Eve Goldberg, Heriberto G., Tim Harrison, Itzamna Jimenez, Les Jones, Shellye Jones, Carole Mitnick, Joey Mogul, Flor Monterrosa, Lui Sanchez, Smitty Smith, Joe Stokes, and Mary, Bryce, and Kaira Danico. I offer special thanks to Itzamna and Crissy for providing valuable insight on several chapters of the book manuscript.

Tori Booker deserves special recognition as the person who has spent the most time on the telephone with me over the past decade. Despite 2,000 miles between us, her "interventions" helped me through times of crisis and stress, her humor made me laugh when I needed it the most, and her copyediting of the first four chapters was exemplary.

I have been extremely lucky to have a biological/legal family that is part of my "family of choice." They have helped guide me through dark valleys and held my hand ascending dazzling peaks. My niece and nephews—Kelsey and Devin MacKenzie and Andres ("Sito") Stockdill Garay—have been a constant source of laughter and pride as well as a source of hope for the future. Thanks to my brother-in-law Mack MacKenzie for summer fun in Colorado and beyond. Thanks to my sister Juli MacKenzie for believing in me throughout my life and showing me, through spirit and example, the importance of perseverance, humor, and independence. I thank my *compita* and sister Flor de Maria Garay (a.k.a. Carla), who has provided me with spiritual solidarity, hours of "cotherapy," and a remarkable example of progressive struggle and defiance. I am also indebted to my brother Darin Stockdill for calling me, taking the time to listen both to my despair and my dreams, encouraging me to persist in my efforts, reading every page at least once, and being with me to blaze paths in the wilderness. Thanks, bro! Finally, I thank my parents Jim and Joyce Stockdill, with all my heart, for encouraging me from an early age to think critically and act with compassion. My parents have read much of my work and offered valuable advice and heartfelt support. I certainly could not have made it this far without the love of my family.

Last of all, I must acknowledge all those individuals who have taught me about the injustices entrenched in our society and challenged me to take part in struggles for change. In addition to the people already mentioned, I thank the dedicated activists of the Free South Africa Coordinating Committee and the United Coalition Against Racism at the University of Michigan, Chicago's Puerto Rican Independence Movement, ACT UP/Chicago, as well as the students of Red Nations and Movimiento Estudiantil Chicano/a de Aztlan (MECHA) at Cal Poly Pomona. The individuals in these organizations and others too countless to name have constantly reminded me of powerful legacies of resistance as well as the hope for a better world.

Although many people have helped me to complete this project, any errors of interpretation or other mistakes are, of course, mine.

—*B. C. S.*

1

AIDS, Multiple Inequalities, and Activism

In the year 2003, we are at a crossroads in the AIDS (acquired immunodeficiency syndrome) crisis. Never before has there been so much promise: We know how to prevent the transmission of HIV (human immunodeficiency virus), and we have the means to do so. We have treatments for fighting both the virus and the opportunistic infections that ravage the bodies of those living with AIDS. At the same time, the institutional bigotry and greed that have marked U.S. society's responses to the crisis since the early 1980s continue—in new and old forms. People are still dying of AIDS. In the United States, HIV infection for men, women, and youth in prison is still often a death sentence. Outside the prison walls, people of color, injection drug users, and poor people in general continue to be infected and die at alarming rates. Black and Latino gay men as well as black* and

*In accordance with the publisher's style, the racial groups designating "black" and "white" are not capitalized in this book. However, I typically capitalize them because I consider the terms to be proper nouns, referring to specific racial groups in the United States and not mere descriptions of skin color. By capitalizing these terms, I do not mean to reify them as biological categories (they are not), but rather to highlight that they are socially constructed categories that exist and affect the quality of life of millions of people. Although fluid and complex, these two racial categories are very real and have significant historical and contemporary meanings. While some choose to capitalize "black" and not "white," I believe that in social science writings it is important to indicate not only oppressed racial groups, but privileged racial groups as well. In the United States, whites collectively comprise the dominant racial group that benefits from the oppression of people of color (see also Rothenberg 2002).

Latina women continue to have disproportionately high infection and death rates. In the third world, the vast majority of the estimated 36 million people with HIV/AIDS (Centers for Disease Control 2001) will undoubtedly die within a few years as multinational pharmaceuticals and the "free trade" organizations that support them persist in their efforts to keep antiviral drugs out of the bodies that need them.

Which road will activists, public health workers, political leaders, and others take? A crucial part of figuring out what directions to take today involves looking back at the lessons of AIDS activism in the not-so-distant past. HIV/AIDS has *always* been a problem that has severely affected those at the intersections of multiple oppressions: homophobia, racism, sexism, and classism in particular. In turn, these same inequalities have been intertwined with collective responses to a disease that has taken approximately 500,000 lives in the United States and over 22 million lives worldwide (Centers for Disease Control 2001). Since 1981, despite rich and critical research possibilities, there has been little sociological research that has focused on the interactions between *multiple* inequalities and AIDS activism. That is not surprising, given that between the years of 1986 and 1999, the *American Sociological Review,* the *Journal of American Sociology,* and *Social Forces* (considered by some to be the most prestigious sociological journals in the United States) published a total of *zero* articles on HIV/AIDS (Lichtenstein 2001).[1] Outside of these mainstream journals, there is a considerable amount of sociological literature on the AIDS crisis, but with a few notable exceptions, minimal attention has been paid to AIDS *activism* (J. Gamson 1989; Epstein 1996; Stoller 1998).[2]

The goal of this book is to help fill in this gap, to explore what has happened at "the intersections" of HIV/AIDS from a sociological perspective. I analyze AIDS activism within the context of interlocking racial, class, gender, and heterosexual oppressions. My analysis is based on multiple research methods, including in-depth interviews with fifty AIDS activists, my own participation in AIDS organizing, organizational documents, and other sources. I examine examples of AIDS activism at the crossroads, where multiple inequalities created both conflicts and cooperation: activism combating HIV/AIDS among not only gay men but also prisoners, people of color, women, and injection drug users—groups that overlap in significant ways. I explore how inequalities have interacted on societal, community, and movement levels to impede activism and how activists have worked to forge more inclusive approaches to fighting AIDS.

Ideological and strategic rifts within the AIDS movement of the late 1980s and early 1990s were often cut along lines of race, class, gender, and sexuality.[3] Internal movement divisions that affected political perspectives and strategies were often influenced by activists' own experiences with inequality (e.g., being a gay male Pacific Islander versus a gay white man), as well as their prior political experience (e.g., being active in the Puerto Rican independence movement versus having no prior activist experience). For example, gay men of color were often at odds with white gay men over how to respond to the impact of racism on the AIDS crisis. ACT UP members with prior progressive or radical political organizing experience were more likely to advocate taking action to provide support to prisoners affected by HIV/AIDS than members with no prior organizing experience, who were often resistant to such efforts. This book analyzes such conflicts as well as strategies to overcome them. Challenging oppressions at multiple levels (personal, community, institutional) has been an essential part of the work of AIDS activists. For me, the most instructive lessons are those involving the creation of (and the obstacles to) more inclusive understandings of the AIDS crisis and more inclusive activist approaches that empower marginalized communities and confront multiple inequalities. For example, one Los Angeles activist spoke about the challenges in providing AIDS-related services to a group of homeless, transgendered, Salvadoran immigrants—a group targeted by several forms of stigma and discrimination. Lessons about such AIDS activism at "the intersections" can optimally be used by activists, policymakers, and scholars to more fully understand and combat HIV/AIDS, as well as myriad other social and public health problems.

Multiple Oppressions and HIV/AIDS

The AIDS movement developed in response to massive death fueled by government, media, and corporate inaction and bigotry in the 1980s. The failure to mount rapid, comprehensive responses to the emerging epidemic in the 1980s was caused in large part by the marginalized position of the vast majority of AIDS victims vis-à-vis systems of inequality (Shilts 1987; Carter 1992; Cohen 1999; Corea 1992; Arno and Feiden 1992; Hammonds 1992; Deresiewicz 1991; see also essays in ACT UP/New York 1992 and McKenzie 1991). A virulent and deadly homophobia, in particular, prompted the earliest negligent and punitive institutional responses in the 1980s (Crimp

1990; Patton 1990). Furthermore, homophobia also blinded society to HIV/AIDS among women and people of color because AIDS was seen as a "gay disease." As the AIDS crisis unfolded, homophobia was soon joined by racism, classism, and sexism.[4] Gay men, injection drug users, people of color, poor people, and women (and people at the intersections of these groups) were dying, and society, for the most part, remained silent. When action was finally taken, the AIDS intervention and prevention efforts of the federal government and other dominant institutions (e.g., the mainstream media and the medical establishment) were by and large woefully inadequate and overdue.

Consequently, AIDS activist campaigns to prevent the spread of HIV, provide services to those living with HIV and AIDS, and galvanize scientific research were forced to confront social inequality. These efforts have included extensive campaigns to transform public consciousness around AIDS and related issues; the formation of AIDS service agencies; negotiations with government bureaucracies to promote access to resources and services; and direct action protests targeting pharmaceuticals, government agencies, the insurance industry, the health care system, and the mass media. Challenging collective values and beliefs that devalue the lives of lesbian, gay, bisexual, and transgendered (LGBT) people, people of color, women, injection drug users, and poor people as well as promoting more humane ways of thinking were crucial movement activities (Corea 1992; Crimp 1990; J. Gamson 1989; Patton 1990; Stoller 1998). Below, I briefly outline how different inequalities have affected the AIDS crisis as well as some of the challenges that have faced AIDS activists in these areas. Although initially presented separately, these oppressions are intersecting, as will be discussed shortly.

Homophobia

More U.S. AIDS deaths have occurred among gay and bisexual men (of all races) than any other group—a fact that is still true today in the third decade of the AIDS crisis (Centers for Disease Control 2001). Looking through the obituary sections of gay and lesbian newspapers in the 1980s and 1990s meant looking at AIDS-related deaths week after week, year after year. According to the Centers for Disease Control, of 774,467 reported cumulative AIDS cases in the United States by the end of 2000, 404,398 (over 52 percent) occurred among *men who have sex with men* (Centers for Disease Control 2001).[5] Homophobia and heterosexism have guided dominant society's responses to AIDS. The perception of AIDS as a monolithically "gay disease" in a homophobic society was central to the failure among many sectors to take adequate action to slow the spread of the disease and educate the public (Shilts 1987; Crimp 1990; Adam 1989; Weeks 1992; Padgug 1989).

Some political and religious leaders constructed AIDS as a punishment for the "perversions" of homosexuality, with gay men portrayed as "carriers" of the deadly scourge—who became villains rather than victims. Robert Padgug (1989) observes that many measures proposed to combat AIDS, such as expulsion, quarantine, mandatory testing, and the removal of PWA (people/person with AIDS) from schools, jobs, and housing, have been patterned on historical forms of homophobic oppression. The hysteria related to AIDS—fueled by the fusion of antigay sentiment, ignorance about HIV/AIDS, and fear of disease—has catalyzed homophobic violence and discrimination targeted at gay men, lesbians, bisexuals, and transgendered people regardless of HIV status. Randy Shilts describes in vivid detail the inaction of the medical profession, scientific research establishments, the mass media, and the federal government, calling the AIDS crisis "a drama of national failure, played out against a backdrop of useless death" (Shilts 1987: xxii).[6]

Institutions (such as gay newspapers and magazines), organizations (e.g., health clinics), and social networks within gay and lesbian communities provided the foundation for the first wave of AIDS activism in the early and mid-1980s (Freedman and D'Emilio 1988; Padgug 1989). People educated each other about AIDS, cared for each other, set up research programs, organized PWA collectives, and demanded increased government research and funding (Arno and Feiden 1992; Stoller 1998). AIDS agencies established within the gay community, such as AIDS Project Los Angeles (APLA) and the Gay Men's Health Crisis (GMHC) in New York City, developed extensive prevention programs and a vast array of medical, psychological, and social services for people living with HIV and AIDS. A crucial element of AIDS services was the formation of emotional support groups to help people with HIV/AIDS deal with psychological trauma precipitated by stigma, isolation, and discrimination. These efforts were hindered by homophobia and heterosexism within the health care system, the legal system, the mass media, the family, and diverse communities. Activists had to convince those in power and the general heterosexual population that gay lives were worth saving and/or force them to take action against the growing tide of AIDS (Crimp 1990; Patton 1990; Carter 1992).[7]

Grieving and frustrated with the lack of progress in fighting the disease, a group of people, many of them living with HIV/AIDS and most of them gay, lesbian, or bisexual, formed the confrontational AIDS Coalition to Unleash Power (ACT UP) in New York City in 1987 (and soon thereafter in numerous cities around the world). ACT UP was self-described this way: "A diverse, nonpartisan group of individuals united in anger and committed to direct action to end the AIDS Crisis. We meet with government and health officials; we research and distribute the latest medical information. We protest and demonstrate; we are not silent" (Carter 1992: 1). Taking to the streets to protest, ACT UP represented the coalescence of "queer" oppositional consciousness (collective beliefs that oppose a system of oppression) as LGBTs increasingly acted upon the realization that their interests were at odds with those of the dominant society. Progressive and radical lesbians, gay men, bisexuals, and transgendered people in ACT UP and other groups such as Queer Nation reclaimed the pejorative term *queer* throughout the 1990s. This term has been consciously used as a way to defy homophobia by embracing sexual "difference," distinct cultural traditions, and political struggles and to be inclusive of not only gay men but also lesbians, bisexuals, and transgendered people (see Crimp 1990; Deitcher 1995).[8]

From 1987 to 1995, ACT UP chapters across the nation used direct action tactics (marches, sit-ins, die-ins, phone and fax zaps) to target exorbitant antiviral drug prices, inadequate government funding for research and prevention, the sluggish pace of HIV/AIDS medical research, inaccessible clinical trials, and other inequities of the epidemic (Carter 1992; Cohen 1998; Arno and Feiden 1992; Gould 2000).[9] Simultaneously, they also challenged cultural norms that condemn homosexuality. This cultural defiance included throwing condoms at public officials (to protest the government's refusal to air advertisements about condom use, a refusal that contributed to unsafe sex and unnecessary deaths), same-sex kissing in public places, speaking explicitly and positively about anal sex, and unfurling banners promoting safer sex at public events. ACT UP's mission to emphasize the value of queer lives and vocally defy the status quo was encapsulated in the slogan "Silence = Death." This powerful slogan appeared on T-shirts, stickers, and posters, along with the symbol of the pink triangle that gay men were forced to wear in Nazi concentration camps during the Holocaust.

ACT UP was primarily a middle-class, white gay male group, but there were smaller numbers of women, people of color, and other social groups active in the organization (Cohen 1998; Gould 2000; Stoller 1998). In turn, the oppositional consciousness symbolized by "Silence = Death" was adopted by other communities, including recovering substance abusers and prisoners. For example, the newsletter of the Prisoners with AIDS Rights Advocacy Group was emblazoned with the pink triangle and the slogan "Silence = Death."[10]

Extensive educational programs and social protest, coupled with underground research and treatment groups as well as more traditional "politicking," have been integral in raising awareness in LGBT communities and broader society, increasing government AIDS budgets, opening up experimental trials, and making treatment more accessible for people with AIDS (Carter 1992; Corea 1992; ACT UP/New York 1992; Arno and Feiden 1992; Cohen 1998). Today, there is a veritable AIDS "industry," with annual expenditures in the billions of dollars, that developed as a result of the angry voices and actions taken since the 1980s.

Sexism

Women AIDS activists have consistently stressed that pervasive gender inequality has increased the threat of HIV/AIDS among women (Anastos and Marte 1991; Hammonds 1992; ACT UP/New York 1992). Particularly in the first years of the epidemic, women were invisible victims of AIDS (Stoller 1998; Corea 1992). The social construction of AIDS as a gay male disease coupled with sexism in the government, the medical establishment, and the larger society served to put women at risk for HIV infection and led to shorter survival times after diagnosis. At the end of 2000, women accounted for approximately 17 percent (130,104) of cumulative AIDS cases in the United States—a percentage that has steadily increased since the 1980s (Centers for Disease Control 2001). Despite the fact that there were women dying of AIDS in the United States in the early 1980s, there was a dearth of medical research on AIDS among women throughout the 1980s and well into the 1990s. As a result, there were few resources available to women, particularly in the 1980s. Women found it difficult to gain access to clinical drug trials and AIDS-related health care in general. Women were implicitly (and sometimes explicitly) told that they were not at risk for HIV infection. These factors led to extreme social isolation for many women living with HIV/AIDS.

Various aspects of patriarchal society made women uniquely vulnerable to HIV/AIDS (ACT UP/New York 1992). Their subordinate positions in heterosexual relationships often put them at risk for HIV infection by way of sexual violence, refusal of men to wear condoms, and the criminalization of prostitution (which makes sex workers more vulnerable to sexual abuse and violence). Their unequal economic status meant that they had less access to quality health care than men. Women's traditional roles call for them to take care of others before they take care of themselves, and their responsibilities as breadwinners, spouses, and mothers often hastened the progression of AIDS. In the face of the impact of HIV/AIDS among women, they were often vilified as "vectors of transmission" (to men and to children) rather than seen as people actually at risk themselves.

Gena Corea (1992) describes how women in ACT UP and other organizations pushed for more research on the effects of AIDS on women (see also ACT UP/New York 1992). Women in ACT UP led several protests, such as disrupting conferences and holding sit-ins at the Centers for Disease Control and Prevention (CDC) to protest its clinical definition of AIDS, which did not include the primary manifestations of AIDS in women until 1993. This definition effectively prevented many women from receiving medical treatment, health and disability benefits, rent subsidies, child care, and other support services. In turn, because relatively few women had been clinically diagnosed with AIDS, the government perceived less need for prevention efforts. Women's caucuses in ACT UP exposed the male bias within the medical establishment (encapsulated in the CDC definition of AIDS) with slogans such as: "Women don't get AIDS. They just die from it." Activists protested at hospitals that failed to provide adequate care for women with AIDS and at media sources that produced inaccurate information on women and AIDS. Women (particularly lesbians) in ACT UP, as well as women in communities of color, often served as bridges between different communities and organizations as they strived to confront not only homophobia but also sexism, racism, and classism related to the AIDS crisis (Stoller 1998).

Women from various communities worked arduously to conduct research, gather and disseminate information, and establish services for women affected by HIV/AIDS. Creating programs for women meant simultaneously reconceptualizing women as whole people rather than solely childbearers and wives, as well as confronting the male-centered health care system. While combating institutional barriers and sexist ideology, women AIDS activists across the country have built a network of health care, emotional support, and various social services for women living with HIV/AIDS. The status of women with HIV/AIDS has improved in recent years, but follow-up discussions with activists indicate that programs for women with HIV/AIDS are still underfunded and that many women with HIV/AIDS remain isolated without access to emotional support, quality health care, and other services.

Racism

People of color, particularly African Americans and Native Americans, have been disproportionately represented among HIV infections and AIDS deaths since the 1980s. For example, by the end of 2000, African Americans accounted for 38 percent of *cumulative* AIDS cases in the United States, though they comprise only about 12.5 percent of the U.S. population. The percentage of reported total AIDS cases among African Americans has increased over the last twenty years. In 1999, 47 percent of *new* AIDS cases were among African Americans. According to the CDC, AIDS was the number one killer of African American men between the ages of twenty-five and forty-four from 1991 through 1998 (Centers for Disease Control 2000a). Latinos/as, who compose approximately 13 percent of the U.S. population, represent 18 percent of cumulative AIDS cases. Asian Americans and Pacific Islanders, who comprise 3.7 percent of the U.S. population, make up about 7 percent of cumulative AIDS cases. Native Americans (including Alaskan Natives), who make up 0.9 percent of the U.S. population, accounted for 3 percent of cumulative AIDS cases, making them the racial group with the highest rate of AIDS (Centers for Disease Control 2001; U.S. Bureau of the Census 2001).[11]

Institutionalized racism in many different forms has exacerbated the AIDS crisis in communities of color. Like women and gay men, people of color affected by HIV/AIDS received inadequate attention by the government, medical researchers, the mass media, and other institutions during the first decade of the AIDS crisis and beyond. Economic injustice and political exclusion targeting communities of color has historically translated into impoverished living conditions, including inferior health care, housing, and education—all of which have made people of color more vulnerable to HIV/AIDS (Cohen 1999; Deresiewicz 1991; Braithwaite and Lythcott 1991).

During the emergence of HIV/AIDS in the United States, the Reagan administration mounted a fierce assault on communities of color. Clarence Lusane (1991) notes that existing social problems, including AIDS, in black and Latino/a communities were intensified by the erosion of civil rights legislation and affirmative action, the entrance of crack cocaine into U.S. cities, and immense cutbacks in social services. Lusane demonstrates the federal government's complicity in the infusion of crack cocaine into inner-city neighborhoods in the 1980s and the simultaneous criminalization of people of color. It is seen vividly in the policies of both the "war on drugs" and the "war on crime," which included racist police brutality (Stockdill

2001b), racial profiling, racially biased mandatory sentencing guidelines, mass incarceration, and the trampling of civil rights during the
reactionary Reagan and George H. W. Bush administrations ("Special
Section" 1998; Reiman 1995). Imprisoning and brutalizing thousands
of people of color, particularly youths, further destabilized and impoverished communities of color (Marable 1991). These developments occurred at the same time that AIDS was striking African
American and other communities of color full force and contributed
to the tragedy of AIDS in these communities. Cathy Cohen writes:
"Reagan's general attack on the budget priorities of the poor and people of color coincided with, and in many cases paved the way for, an
underfunding of AIDS" (1999: 83–84).

The mass media more often than not ignored the AIDS crisis in
black and Latino/a communities, rendering people with HIV/AIDS
invisible. The coverage that did appear focused either on "respectful"
victims (e.g., Magic Johnson) or implicitly "immoral" victims (e.g.,
poor addicts). Racially biased images in the media often sent out the
message that people of color, especially poor people of color, were
among the "dispensable" victims of AIDS (Patton 1990; Carter 1992;
Hammonds 1992). Cohen's (1999) research sheds light on the multiple hierarchies of HIV/AIDS that determine who is "deserving" of
compassion in the eyes of both dominant white institutions and organizations (e.g., the *New York Times*) and middle- and upper-class
black institutions and organizations (e.g., *Ebony* magazine). She
shows that African American gay men, injection drug users, and poor
women have frequently been blamed or overlooked rather than supported during the AIDS crisis.

Activists in communities of color found that in order to fight
AIDS, they had to fight systemic exclusion, challenge dehumanizing
collective beliefs, and transform collective identities. AIDS activists
of color have had to struggle just to demonstrate the gravity of the
AIDS crisis in their communities and to acquire funds to initiate
AIDS programs and services (Cohen 1999). Community-based AIDS
agencies serving communities of color have been consistently underfunded by the government and other sources (Dalton 1991; Deresiewicz 1991; Levenson 2000). In addition to securing funds, activists
have had to address the public prejudice and severely restricted access to health care and other services facing poor people of color and
other marginalized groups (Saalfield 1992; Christensen 1992; Stoller
1998; Farmer 1996). Complex issues linked to poverty—housing,
welfare, substance abuse, incarceration, and violence—have all been
issues that AIDS activists have had to deal with on a daily basis in

many communities of color. Furthermore, many activists of color—in particular, Latinos/as and Asian Americans—face the challenges of working with immigrant populations, which are often targets of discrimination because of language barriers and "legal status."

The struggle to establish AIDS-related social and health services for people of color has been an extremely difficult one. In many cities, mega-agencies like GMHC and APLA have created more inclusive programs for people of color. At the same time, community-based agencies and programs (e.g., the Minority AIDS Project in Los Angeles and the Kupona Network in Chicago) for people of color have been established in various cities across the country. Although there are more services and programs for people of color today, communities of color continue to be disproportionately affected by HIV/AIDS as a result of the continued racism embodied in the decimation of welfare by the Welfare Reform Act of 1996, anti-immigrant policies, and the continued prioritization of corporate and military spending over health and social services. Today, a central task is to create holistic approaches that address not only HIV/AIDS but also the other complex social and health problems endemic to a racist society.

Classism

ACT UP/New York writes: "In addition to the issue of unequal access to treatment, this country's response to the AIDS crisis in general is profoundly influenced by its class structure and its profit driven economy" (ACT UP/New York 1992: 10). The social problems connected to poverty mentioned in the above sections shaped the experiences of poor people in general—women, men, children, people of color, and whites—within the context of HIV/AIDS. These social problems disproportionately affect the poor and increase their chances of being infected with HIV and developing AIDS (Farmer 1996). Poor people lack access to decent health care, which should include meaningful AIDS prevention messages as well as quality HIV/AIDS-related medical care. They live in substandard housing and sometime on the streets, which increases the risk of health problems in general. In 1992, George Carter noted that there were at least 35,000 homeless people with AIDS in the United States. Drug addiction is another social problem that fuels AIDS in poor communities. Robert Fullilove writes:

> Urban poverty in the United States has created the perfect machinery for the continued propagation of HIV. Inner city poor neighborhoods

often shelter a vigorous drug trade, numerous opportunities for
strangers to engage in drug-mediated, unprotected sex, and numerous locations where these and other risk behaviors go virtually unchallenged. (Fullilove 1995: 96)

Although statistics on socioeconomic status and HIV/AIDS are
often difficult to gather, it is documented that working-class and poor
people have higher rates of HIV infection, AIDS diagnoses, and
deaths than those in the middle and upper classes (ACT UP/New
York 1992; Corea 1992; Farmer 1996). Poor people have less access
to quality AIDS-related programs and services. Research and clinical
drug trials have generally focused on middle- and upper-class people,
in large part because poor people are less likely to have regular contact with doctors who are infectious disease specialists and less able
to fully participate in complicated research studies (Patton 1990;
Stoller 1998). The more than 40 million people without health insurance in the United States are particularly susceptible to HIV/AIDS
because of their lack of access to health care (Carter 1992). Along
with the exorbitant costs of antiviral drugs, these and other factors related to class often spell out catastrophe for poor people living with
HIV/AIDS. Furthermore, many middle-class and working-class people with AIDS experience downward economic mobility; many of
them end up on welfare or disability or both.

AIDS activists in various communities have had to deal with the
thorny issues of class, particularly in communities that are also disproportionately poor—prisoners, women, and people of color (Cohen
1999; Corea 1992). Activists working in the areas of welfare rights,
homelessness, and addiction have increasingly had to take on the
AIDS crisis (Stoller 1998). Although clean needle exchange programs and HIV/AIDS programs for prisoners have been developed in
various locations, these programs consistently face the problem of
scarce funding and lack of popular support. Activists have had to
challenge class-based structural inequities (e.g., large cuts in government health care spending) and prejudice (e.g., stigma targeting welfare recipients) as AIDS-related deaths continue to rise. They have
also worked to counter the facts that AIDS as an economic issue has
seldom been covered by the mass media and that federal spending for
social services has been consistently cut since the 1980s.

The Intersections of Oppressions

Although the AIDS crisis provides an opportunity to study singular
forms of oppression and their relationships to collective action, the

goal of this book is to analyze the interconnectedness of multiple op-pressions within the context of activism. The above discussion on in-equality and AIDS highlights some of the systematic inequalities interwoven with the AIDS crisis. Racism, sexism, homophobia, and classism, however, do not operate in isolation (Smith 1983; Davis 1983; Collins 1990). Within the context of the AIDS crisis, these forms of oppression often intersect and occur simultaneously. Aca-demic and public policy analyses that fail to examine AIDS within the context of interlocking inequalities that operate on multiple lev-els (family, community, institutional) do not capture the complexity of the AIDS crisis.

HIV infection and AIDS fatality rates among those at the inter-sections of two or more forms of inequality, particularly gay and bi-sexual men of color and women of color, *have always been* and con-tinue to be disproportionately high. The media has trumpeted a shift in HIV/AIDS from the "gay community" to "communities of color" in recent years, but people of color have always been overrepresented in the ranks of those living with and dying of AIDS. Reporting on the alleged shift from "gay" to "of color" also reflects the dangerous false dichotomy of race and sexuality, ignoring the fact that black and Latino gay and bisexual men have suffered the highest rates of HIV infection and AIDS since the early 1980s. The late black gay ac-tivist, poet, and PWA Essex Hemphill wrote more than a decade ago: "Black men suffer a disproportionate number of AIDS deaths in com-munities with very sophisticated gay health services" (Hemphill 1991: xx). In 1993, the CDC reported that there were more than 61,700 diagnosed cases of AIDS among gay and bisexual men of color, accounting for an enormously disproportionate 20 percent of all cumulative cases of AIDS through June 30, 1993 (Centers for Disease Control 1993).[12] In an article entitled "Researchers Raise Concerns on HIV Rate," by Thomas H. Maugh II, the *Los Angeles Times* (February 6, 2001) reported on a 2000 CDC study of 2,400 gay and bisexual men aged twenty-three to twenty-nine in six major U.S. cities. The CDC found that an alarming 12 percent of the men inter-viewed were infected with HIV. As seen in Table 1.1, young African American and Latino gay and bisexual men in the study had HIV in-fection rates respectively over four and two times higher than young white gay men.

Of the young black gay men included in the study, 30 percent were infected with HIV. One can only imagine the outcry by govern-ment officials and the media if 30 percent of young white heterosex-ual men were infected with HIV. I have never seen statistics compar-ing the percentage of gay men (of any race) living with HIV or AIDS

Table 1.1   HIV Infection Rates for Gay and Bisexual Men Aged 23–29,
in Six Major U.S. Cities

Race	Percentage Infected with HIV
White	7
Asian American	5
Pacific Islander	7
Latino	15
African American	30

Source: Thomas H. Maugh II, "Researchers Raise Concerns on HIV Rate," *Los Angeles Times,* February 6, 2001, p. A1.

with their proportion of the larger population. A brief estimation for African American gay men is instructive. African Americans comprised about 12.5 percent of the U.S. population but accounted for 47 percent of new AIDS cases reported in 1999 (21,900 out of 46,400). Approximately half of the new AIDS cases in African Americans were among "men who have sex with men"—representing an alarming *23 percent of all new AIDS cases* (Centers for Disease Control 2000a)—alarming because African American gay men comprise an estimated 0.6 percent of the U.S. population and arguably comprise the majority of black "men who have sex with men."[13]

These rates are linked to the compounded effects of multiple oppressions for gay and bisexual men of color (Cohen 1999; Julien and Mercer 1991; Dalton 1991). Gay and bisexual men of color face the various manifestations of racism, homophobia, and in many cases classism. For example, particularly in the 1980s, AIDS prevention funding specifically for gay men of color was minuscule. Gay and bisexual men of color are less likely to have access to health care (doctors, insurance, clinical trials, antiviral drugs) and AIDS-related services than middle-class white gay men (Tagle 1993). Although drug addiction rates are similar across racial lines, the impact of addiction weighs more heavily on people of color (because they have less access to rehabilitation programs), and untreated addiction increases the likelihood not only of HIV infection but progression to full-blown AIDS (Lusane 1991). Gay men of color face alienation and stigma in both communities of color and in gay communities, fostering isolation and making it extremely difficult for them to find support (Beam 1986; Hemphill 1991).

In 1992, Marion Banzhaf reported that 73 percent of all women with AIDS in the United States were women of color, although they comprised only about 25 percent of all women. Although other women of color have disproportionately high rates of AIDS, African American women continue to have the highest rates among women. In 1999, 63 percent *of all women* with AIDS were African American. In 1996, African American women comprised about 12 percent of new AIDS cases (including men and women)—double their proportion (approximately 6 percent) in the general population (Centers for Disease Control 1998).

Evelynn Hammonds writes that "only a multi-faceted African American feminist analysis attentive to issues of race, sex, gender and power can adequately expose the impact of AIDS in our communities and formulate just policies to save women's lives" (Hammonds 1992: 22). As with gay men of color, disproportionately high AIDS rates among women of color are related to multiple inequalities linked to their lack of access to meaningful prevention messages, health care, and support systems (Cohen 1999; Farmer 1996; Hammonds 1992; Banzhaf 1992). Male dominance in heterosexual relationships often places women of color at risk for unsafe sex. Poverty makes many women of color vulnerable to risky behaviors such as trading unsafe sex for drugs or money. Paul Farmer describes the systemic assaults on Darlene, an African American woman living in Harlem:

> As a heroin user, a habit clearly tied to a poverty structured by racism, her chances of avoiding HIV were slim, even if she had wanted to quit prior to her diagnosis. In 1987, the year that Darlene's world was burst asunder by AIDS, there were 338,365 treatment slots available to the nation's four million addicts, and most of these programs predominantly served men. As a pregnant woman, Darlene would have found it next to impossible to find treatment for her addiction. (Farmer 1996: 20–21)

Other groups, such as prisoners and injection drug users, are frequently subject to what sociologist Deborah King (1988) terms "double jeopardy" (and, in many cases, triple jeopardy). Most prisoners are poor or working class and disproportionately black and Latino/a and thus face classism and racism ("Special Section" 1998). LGBT prisoners face homophobia, and female prisoners face sexism. Injection drug users come from all racial and class backgrounds, but, as Lusane (1991) points out, poor people of color face more severe consequences for addiction and find fewer resources for rehabilitation, which has direct implications for HIV infection and AIDS. Prisoners and injection drug users have disproportionately high HIV infection and AIDS death rates when compared to the general population (Stockdill 1995; Saalfield 1992).

* * *

Each of the above inequalities, as well as others not discussed here, merits more extensive discussion. For example, several activists discussed ableism—discrimination and prejudice targeting differently abled people (often referred to as "physically disabled"). Jeff, an Asian American–Pacific Islander gay activist, stated that there is a "need to see differently abled people as part of the whole." Although this examination of the AIDS crisis and inequality is, out of necessity, a brief overview, the importance of enhancing our understanding of how movement dynamics are shaped by multiple forms of oppression is, I hope, clear.

Social Movement Theory

In terms of social movement theory, my goals are twofold.[14] First, I hope to build upon the limited social movement scholarship on AIDS activism. Second, using the case of the AIDS movement, I hope to demonstrate the critical importance of analyzing how multiple, interlocking oppressions affect collective action.

Currently, social movement scholars are exploring the links between culture (identity, consciousness, symbolic meanings) and structure (organizations, networks, institutional policies and practices) within the context of collective action. Challenging "classical" collective behavior theories that lumped social movements into the same category as fads, hysterias, trends, and panics, "resource mobilization" models, based on research on movements of the 1960s, demonstrate that movements are grounded in preexisting organizations, institutions, and social networks (Morris and Herring 1987; McAdam, McCarthy, and Zald 1988). These forms of social organization facilitate the mobilization of resources (money, meeting places, communication technologies, labor) that are employed in the political arena to advance group interests. The resource mobilization approach emphasizes the centrality of strategic and tactical choices in determining outcomes.[15]

Although resource mobilization models effectively highlight the structural and organizational forces shaping social movements, they fall short in addressing how these forces interact with culture, collective consciousness, and individual identity. Structural approaches tend to focus only on periods of direct action, thereby neglecting the question of how social movement actors translate discontent into oppositional consciousness and, in turn, channel this consciousness into collective action. Social psychological theories explore how individual commitment to a cause or organization is generated and what makes people act on this commitment, linking micro (individual) and macro (institutional) levels of social movements (Klandermans 1988; W. Gamson 1989; Snow et al. 1986; Snow and Benford 1988; see also essays in Morris and Mueller 1992).[16]

Drawing on Marxist theory, contemporary theoretical models emphasize the critical importance of collective consciousness in social movement development. Collective consciousness refers to a set of beliefs held in common by a group of people. It provides people with a framework used to make sense of their society or world as well as their own experiences. Bert Klandermans (1992) stresses that social-movement activists by necessity challenge dominant collective beliefs and reframe collective perceptions of social relationships in terms of injustice and inequality. For example, in the 1950s, the Mattachine Society helped many gays to reconceptualize their individual experiences of suffering in terms of being members of a culturally and politically oppressed group (D'Emilio 1983). This active process of promoting an oppositional consciousness is central to the development of strategies to fight oppression. In recent decades, African American activists have challenged the notion that high poverty rates stem from dysfunctional (or even pathological) black families and communities that lack "family values," self-discipline, and so on. Instead, they argue that the root causes of African American poverty lie in institutionalized racism manifested in inferior schools, housing, health care, and job opportunities (Davis 1983; Marable 1983).[17]

The transformation of collective consciousness is a crucial aspect of social movement development: people in marginalized groups must be able to see their situation as shared before they can collectively challenge both cultural and institutional domination (Gamson 1992; Taylor and Whittier 1992). For example, social movement organizations frequently use cultural symbols to involve people in collective action, attempting to root their messages in the collective beliefs of target groups (e.g., the use of biblical references by black ministers to encourage involvement in the Civil Rights movement).[18]

Carol Mueller (1992) and Aldon Morris (1992) argue that we must analyze how systematic inequalities affect the consciousness, culture, organizations, and strategies of communities engaging in social protest. From this perspective, the social movement organization serves as a mediator between the broader social and political environment and the mobilization of resources at the individual level, attempting to transform collective identities and beliefs. A key factor in fostering oppositional consciousness is the *social location* of movement participants. Contemporary social psychological theorists view the social movement actor as "socially embedded," examining how the social location of the participant (e.g., an activist's experiences as a Native American woman) shapes her interpretation of grievances as well as the availability of resources and opportunities (Mueller 1992).[19]

However, minimal research has been conducted on how people are drawn into collective action within the context of *multiple* oppressions and *multiple* consciousnesses. How does the interaction of interlocking inequalities affect the emergence and development of activism? For example, how does the political consciousness of a poor Asian American woman differ from that of an upper-class Asian American man? How are mobilization and strategies affected by multiple oppressions? Most sociological research on social movements has focused on consciousness raising and collective action targeting one particular form of social inequality—neglecting collective consciousness and action that seeks to transform more than one system of domination.[20] Morris observes that much sociological scholarship is "likely to overlook the centrality of multiple consciousnesses and interlocking systems of human domination and how they affect collective action" (Morris 1992: 362).

Lessons from Black Feminist Theory

Even as mainstream sociologists and other social scientists have typically examined structural inequalities in isolation, a central tenet of black feminist theory is that classism, racism, sexism, and heterosexism are mutually reinforcing systems of inequality (Combahee River Collective 1983; Smith 1983; Davis 1983; Lorde 1984). Black feminist theory (as well as critical feminist theory developed by other women of color and white lesbians) was developed in the 1970s largely in response to the failure of many social movements to be inclusive of race, class, gender, *and* sexuality.[21]

Analyses of interlocking oppressions by feminists of color have illuminated the dynamic of the oppressed as the oppressor, such as when white women are racist or men of color are sexist (see essays in Smith 1983; Anzaldúa and Moraga 1983; Anzaldúa 1990). Morris

(1992) has written about this dynamic from a social movement theory perspective, coining the term *partial oppositional consciousness*. Echoing the work of feminists of color, he argues that "those oppressed by one system of domination may in fact enjoy a position of privilege and power in another" (Morris 1992: 364). This dynamic is expressed in social movements as ideology and strategies that challenge one particular inequality but promote other inequalities. Two of the most commonly cited examples of partial oppositional consciousness are sexism within the Civil Rights and black power movements and racism in the women's movement (Giddings 1984).

Many activists and scholars, especially feminists of color, argue that by targeting only one oppressive system and often actively promoting other systems of oppression, oppositional movements have alienated those at the crossroads of multiple inequalities and severely reduced their potential to transform society (Clarke 1983; Perez 1991; Cameron 1983). Social movements characterized by partial oppositional consciousness have tended to target only one form of oppression, thereby leaving other systems of domination unchallenged. Hegemonic (dominant) consciousness, which supports all systems of oppression, seldom comes "under total attack," according to Morris (1992: 364). Many activists situated at the intersections of multiple inequalities have called for a unified, broad-based battle against the complex set of social structures that sustain race, class, gender, and heterosexual oppression. By necessity, these activists have had to confront multiple oppressions, and many have struggled within movements to create more inclusive oppositional strategies. The Combahee River Collective, a collective of black feminists, issued a statement in 1977 stating that "we are actively committed to struggling against racial, sexual, heterosexual, and class oppression and see as our particular task the development of integrated analysis and practice based upon the fact that the major systems of oppression are interlocking" (Combahee River Collective 1983: 272). Social movement scholars have, by and large, been slow to examine this conceptual framework, but activists from diverse communities have articulated political consciousnesses attentive to interlocking inequalities. In addition to black feminists, other feminists of color (see essays in Trujillo 1991), progressive black gay men (Beam 1986; Hemphill 1991; Riggs 1989), and white lesbian feminists (Rich 1986; Bulkin, Pratt, and Smith 1988; Kaye-Kantrowitz 1989; ACT UP/New York 1992) have put forth a variety of multidimensional analyses and strategies applied in numerous political struggles (e.g., expanding reproductive rights activism to include not only a woman's right to choose to have an abortion but also the issue of sterilization abuse, which dispropor-tionately affects poor women of color).[22] In recent years, these strug-gles have increasingly included the fight against AIDS.

Methodology and Data

The AIDS movement provides rich case studies for investigating the interaction of multiple inequalities and collective action. At this point, it is important to address the question of what is meant by the term *AIDS movement*. Aldon Morris and Cedric Herring examine dif-ferent conceptions of social movements as articulated by different theoretical positions (Marxian, Weberian, collective behavior, re-source mobilization) and conclude: "No definition of social move-ment enjoys a scholarly consensus and there probably will never be such a definition because definitions inevitably reflect the theoretical assumptions of the theorists" (Morris and Herring 1987: 139). Doug McAdam, John McCarthy, and Mayer Zald (1988) acknowledge the broad range of phenomena—public interest lobbies, revolutions, reli-gious movements—that are sometimes lumped together in the cate-gory of social movements. However, their review of social move-ment scholarship focuses on political reform movements, defin-ing social movements as "politics by other means" and thus outside conventional political channels (McAdam, McCarthy, and Zald 1988: 699).

This definition is useful in classifying the AIDS movement. I char-acterize it—specifically during the late 1980s and early 1990s—as a movement because it was composed of a diverse set of people whose needs were not met by existing dominant institutions, such as the gov-ernment, the medical establishment, and pharmaceutical corpora-tions, and who used "politics by other means" to further their collec-tive interests. This collective action included documentation of the impact of HIV/AIDS; "underground" clinical research; buyer's clubs; PWA collectives; community and peer education; marches, rallies, sit-ins, and other protests; video and art projects; press releases ex-posing government inaction; activist conferences; confrontations with public officials; clean needle exchanges; and community-based client advocacy and services.[23] My purpose here is not to delineate the exact boundaries of the AIDS movement, but rather to examine the relationships between different activists and organizations fight-ing the AIDS crisis. Though the borders of the movement were blurred and there was often no clear consensus regarding goals and strategies (as is the case in many social movements), different parts of the movement were aware of one another and took each other into account as they struggled to change society's response to HIV/AIDS (see Appendix A).

For the purposes of this book, I define the AIDS movement as the sum total of different HIV/AIDS organizations during the late 1980s and early 1990s. They include AIDS prevention groups (e.g., AIDS Prevention Team, Los Angeles), community clinics for people living with HIV/AIDS (Howard Brown Memorial Clinic, Chicago), AIDS direct service agencies (e.g., Chicago Women's AIDS Project), information distributing groups (e.g., Project Inform), advocacy groups focusing on HIV/AIDS issues (e.g., AIDS in Prison Project, New York City), and direct action groups (e.g., ACT UP) during the period of study. As I examine the relationships between different segments of the movement as well as internal organizational dynamics, I pay particular attention to activism targeting AIDS among women, prisoners, injection drug users, and people of color. These populations have tended to receive less attention from researchers and less support from the government, mass media, and large AIDS agencies than middle-class white gay men. Activists organizing in these communities have been more likely to grapple with the impact of multiple oppressions on the AIDS crisis.

I employed multiple methods in conducting my research. These methods included interviews with fifty AIDS activists, participant observation in ACT UP/Chicago, and analysis of organizational documents. The data were collected from a diverse set of AIDS activists and organizations, including mainstream agencies serving primarily middle-class white gay communities; ACT UP; and smaller grassroots groups targeting AIDS among prisoners, injection drug users, people of color, and women.

I conducted fifty face-to-face in-depth interviews with AIDS activists in Chicago, Los Angeles, and New York in 1993 and 1994.[24] The respondents included thirty men and twenty women; forty-two lesbians, gay men, and bisexuals and eight heterosexuals; sixteen whites, fifteen African Americans, ten Latinos/as, six Asian Americans and Pacific Islanders, one Native American, and two biracial activists (one Asian American and Native American and one Filipino and African American). The interview (see Appendix B) consists of a set of open-ended questions on the AIDS crisis and AIDS activism. The interviews typically lasted from one to two hours in length. Follow-up phone interviews were conducted with several respondents. Most initial contacts with respondents were made through activist networks developed in my own political work. Other contacts were made through interview respondents who referred me to other activists. Pseudonyms are used to maintain confidentiality.

I engaged in participant observation in the Chicago chapter of ACT UP from 1992 through 1995. This involved going to bimonthly general meetings, committee meetings, rallies, and direct action protests. In particular, I was an active participant in ACT UP/Chicago's Prison Issues Committee and Legal Defense Committee, establishing contact with prisoners, doing research on prison AIDS policies and practices, and helping to organize and implement direct action protests.

The interviews and participant observation were supplemented by various other sources of data, including the analysis of documents from AIDS organizations from around the country (see Appendix A). These documents include outreach materials, mission statements, internal memoranda, position papers, newsletters, and annual reports. Additional data were gathered from government agency reports and memoranda, letters and grievance forms written by prisoners, documentary films, various AIDS-related publications, gay and lesbian newspapers, and attendance at numerous AIDS-related events.

Although analysis of these activists, organizations, and other sources in no way represents a comprehensive treatment of the AIDS movement, they do allow an in-depth look at some crucial aspects of the movement. The interviews and other sources provide data from men and women; gay men, lesbians, bisexuals, and heterosexuals; HIV-positive and HIV-negative people; five different racial groups (African Americans, Asian Americans, Latinos/as, Native Americans, and whites); three major cities; and both service providers and direct action groups.

The Outline of the Book

Given the interplay of multiple oppressions at both the ideological and institutional levels in the AIDS crisis and the lack of social movement research focusing on such interactions, analysis of the AIDS movement provides the opportunity to explore uncharted sociological territory. Focusing on several segments of the AIDS movement, I examine how multiple oppressions shape political consciousness, mobilization, strategies and tactics, alliances, and repression. Using an intersectional approach, I explore not only how race, class, gender, and sexuality divide organizations and communities, but also how activists respond to these divisions and work to forge coalitions of unity both within and between different marginalized communities and organizations. Such dynamics are not visible if one looks at social movement activity through a unidimensional lens that limits analysis to one form of oppression.

In Chapter 2, I lay out the divergent ideological perspectives that characterized different AIDS organizations and activists. Prior activist experience as well as gender are associated with more inclusive political consciousness. Ideological differences are translated into internal movement divisions and conflict—particularly around race, class, gender, and sexuality. Using Morris's (1992) concept of partial oppositional consciousness, I examine how various strains of dominant, or hegemonic, consciousness within oppressed communities and within organizations operated as obstacles to AIDS prevention and intervention. In addition, I analyze different conceptions of "activism" and how these conceptions relate to different ideological stances and strategic choices.

I discuss the strategies developed to combat AIDS in communities of color, primarily by lesbians and gay men of color, in Chapter 3. I argue that partial oppositional consciousness necessitates community-level activism, as well as direct confrontation of elites. In this chapter, I present a picture of activism guided by mobilization strategies such as constructive dialogue, empowerment initiatives, community immersion, and use of cultural traditions. These strategies were designed to challenge community-level inequalities and prejudice that facilitate the spread of the disease and prevent political unity on a larger level. Lesbians and gay male activists of color paid particular attention to the social position of potential participants and utilized racial oppositional consciousness to promote other forms of oppositional consciousness (e.g., gay and lesbian consciousness) and mobilize people to take action against the AIDS crisis.

In Chapter 4, I analyze the efforts of ACT UP/Chicago's Prison Issues Committee to improve AIDS services in Illinois state prisons. This chapter illustrates how certain spheres of activism, in this case prison issues, were marginalized within the larger AIDS movement. Dominant perceptions of prisoners stymied organizational efforts and necessitated campaigns to humanize prisoners. In turn, the conditions of incarceration created barriers to outside activists attempting to work with prisoners. I flesh out the multiple fronts of social movement activity around AIDS in prison, including extensive research work and efforts to transform public consciousness that serve as key building blocks for direct action tactics. More specifically, activists in this area worked to expand oppositional consciousness to be more inclusive of racial and class issues related to incarceration.

How repression affected the AIDS movement within the context of multiple oppressions is the subject of Chapter 5. In communities of color, fear of repression had a chilling effect on collective action. Many activists were aware of the widespread repression perpetrated by local police forces and the federal government (particularly the Federal Bureau of Investigation) against leftist movements in the 1960s and 1970s. This knowledge, coupled with the threat of contemporary police brutality and racism in the criminal justice system, diminished the prospect of employing confrontational protest methods. In turn, ACT UP members were targeted by police brutality, criminal prosecution, and government surveillance. This repression was one factor in the demise of many ACT UP chapters. I argue that the fear of repression in communities of color, coupled with actual repression targeting ACT UP, inhibited possible coalition building between organizations and communities.

The empirical and theoretical questions raised here are by no means distinct to the AIDS movement. In Chapter 6, I synthesize the primary findings of the preceding chapters and their relevance for social movement theory. I outline five propositions on the dynamic relationships among systemic oppression, political consciousness, and social movements. Central to these propositions is the importance of developing an *intersectional* theoretical framework, one that is attentive to multiple, interlocking systems of inequality. Just as the AIDS crisis can be viewed as a microcosm of the interlocking inequalities that shape different social problems, the AIDS movement provides a laboratory for studying the multiple, often conflicting, streams of consciousness and collective responses that are present in many social movements. A close investigation of the AIDS movement is particularly useful because it raises these issues in sharp detail. Finally, I present important lessons gleaned from my analysis that can be applied not only by AIDS activists but also by activists and policymakers working to combat other social problems.

2

Framing the AIDS Crisis: Inequalities and Divisions on the Movement and Community Levels

You may be surprised to know that the menace is not, in my view, AIDS itself, or HIV. . . . What is more threatening to our community is what lesbian activist Amber Holibaugh so appropriately named her video, "The Second Epidemic." This is an epidemic of discrimination, fear, bigotry and homophobia which will certainly damage the Latino communities in a way that will have deeper effects than HIV ever can.

—Raymond Navarro (1991),
activist, videomaker, writer, and PWA

How have activists framed the "Second Epidemic"? In what ways has it extended into the consciousness of communities themselves? Ideology and collective consciousness are crucial aspects of social movement development (Morris and Herring 1987; McAdam, McCarthy, and Zald 1988). Dominant consciousness serves to legitimate existing patterns of inequality, whereas oppositional consciousness provides the ideological foundation for challenges to oppressive social systems (Gramsci 1987; Marx 1977; Roscigno 1994). Although some social movement scholars have examined the development of oppositional consciousness (Fantasia 1989; Piven and Cloward 1977; Adam 1987), there has been little scholarship on how multiple forms of inequality affect the transformation of consciousness and mobilization (Morris 1992). One notable exception is political scientist

Cathy Cohen's cogent analysis of responses to HIV/AIDS in African American communities. Cohen stresses that these responses have been shaped not only by racism and other inequalities emanating from dominant society but by classism, homophobia, and sexism within black communities themselves:

> While multiple identities are not only recognized but increasingly play a significant role in structuring the lived experience of black people, many community organizations and leaders seem determined to espouse a politics rooted in a unidimensional understanding of racial identity, where the status of middle-class, male or heterosexual provides privilege and attention. (Cohen 1999: 19)

The tension between multidimensional and unidimensional consciousnesses, on the interrelated levels of community and social movement, is the topic of this chapter. More specifically, I examine the predictors of oppositional AIDS consciousness and lay out a continuum of ideological AIDS "frames" (collective perceptions of social problems and possible strategies for change) found among AIDS activists. Expressions of partial oppositional consciousness (ideologies and strategies that challenge one form of inequality but not other forms) within the AIDS movement are described and analyzed. Finally, contested definitions of oppositional consciousness are presented and dissected. The aim of this analysis is to expand our knowledge of how interlocking oppressions are manifested in divergent streams of political consciousness that in turn affect internal organizational dynamics, strategies, tactics, and relationships between groups.

AIDS Consciousness

> Radically different metaphors of power, of community, of resistance are deployed across different sites in the class war surrounding AIDS. . . . Representation of AIDS at every level—in the media, in the science, in the cultural assumptions manifest in the effects of institutional process—are multiple and discontinuous. (Patton 1990: 1)

Collective beliefs about the AIDS crisis are extremely diverse. In the eyes of some, AIDS is a punishment for sin and immorality. For others, AIDS is perceived as a genocidal government plot targeting people of color and/or gays. As discussed in Chapter 1, the AIDS crisis has been inextricably intertwined with multiple inequalities. Thus, how individuals, including activists, frame the AIDS crisis in their minds depends in large part on their understandings of systemic oppression. Although consciousness about AIDS cannot be neatly compartmentalized into two separate ideological boxes marked "hegemonic" (dominant beliefs supporting inequality) and "oppositional" (beliefs challenging inequality), it is possible to delineate major ideological frames that have been central in shaping responses to the AIDS crisis.

Homophobia has been at the core of dominant AIDS ideology from the outset: "All of the dominant discourse on AIDS has encoded the homosexual Other" (Patton 1990: 127). Along with gays, injection drug users, prisoners, and poor people have been seen by many as deserving of the illness or at least not worthy of an all-out effort to fight the fatal disease (Crimp 1990; Stockdill 1995; Saalfield 1992; Carter 1992). AIDS discourse has often been cloaked in moral terms, with the virus as a punishment for sin, crime, or pathology (Padgug 1989; Weeks 1992). At the same time, hegemonic AIDS discourse has been masked by (allegedly) "objective" and "neutral" science (Epstein 1996). The portrayal of AIDS as a purely scientific, medical phenomenon obscured the role of prejudice and discrimination in fueling its spread.

In response to victim blaming and elite inaction in the face of death, people with HIV/AIDS and their allies actively challenged dominant ideology (Gould 2000). This oppositional consciousness and action defied collective beliefs that accept the expertise of medical authorities and condemn gay men and lesbians as inferior. AIDS activists asserted that people with AIDS should be active participants in their own health care, that "queer" is good, and that "Silence = Death." Patton writes that "people living with AIDS would not stay quiet for long. Their discourse shifted to a critique of the oppression of early death and unnecessary infection resulting from treatments delayed and education denied" (Patton 1990: 130). Consciousness around AIDS coalesced into lesbian and gay (later termed *queer*) consciousness (Ames, Atchinson, and Rose 1994; J. Gamson 1989; Crimp 1990; Gould 2000), feminist consciousness (Corea 1992; ACT UP/New York 1992; Hammonds 1992), and antiracist consciousness (Cohen 1999; Hemphill 1991; see also Chapter 3). AIDS consciousness is not expressed in the same ways within different communities and groups. However, at a minimum, we can define AIDS consciousness as a recognition that prejudice and institutional inequality have exacerbated the impact of AIDS and a collective belief that people living with HIV and AIDS are deserving of compassion, health care, and social support rather than stigmatization and discrimination.

What are the predictors of a basic level of AIDS consciousness— a feeling that something was (and is) *fundamentally wrong* with society's response to the epidemic and that something should be done about it? The interviews and participant observation for this study indicate that there were two primary factors associated with individuals becoming AIDS activists: prior involvement in liberal, progressive, or radical social change activities and being personally affected by HIV/AIDS.

Echoing findings for other movements, the majority of activists interviewed for this study were immersed in political networks prior to doing AIDS work (McAdam 1988; Freeman 1973), including involvement in explicitly leftist politics, broad-based reform movements of the 1960s and 1970s, campus activism, Latin American and antiapartheid solidarity work, and advocacy work within liberal social service agencies.[1] In many cases, this activism was driven by the respondents' personal experiences and identities as people of color, women, gay men, bisexuals, and lesbians. For example, Tyrone, a black gay activist in Los Angeles, stated that he was "active from day one in the African American community" and listed more than half a dozen black organizations in which he was involved, including the National Association for the Advancement of Colored People (NAACP) and the Urban League. Later on in his life, he became increasingly involved in gay organizations as well as AIDS organizations, including the Black Coalition on AIDS in San Francisco and the Gay Men of Color Consortium in Los Angeles. Thus, activists' social positions (in relation to systems of inequality) were intertwined with their activist paths.

For a small number of interview respondents, a combination of social consciousness and career opportunities led to AIDS work. Catalina, a Latina active in feminist and antiracist struggles, applied for positions in several social service agencies and accepted a job at a Detroit AIDS organization. Her work as a case manager was shaped by her ideological background in other movements. Kristine, a white lesbian, became involved with the AIDS Foundation of Chicago after a long history of working for feminist advocacy groups. Brent, a gay white man in Chicago, was drawn into AIDS legal advocacy because of personal ties to the gay community and his work as a lawyer for other social causes.

The disruption and loss caused by the disease itself was a second factor in predicting AIDS consciousness; mass illness and death sparked collective action. For several respondents, finding out that they were HIV-positive was also a catalyst for activism. They felt the sting of bigotry, experienced firsthand the lack of government action, and felt compelled to take action. Many of the interview respondents became involved in AIDS activism after finding out that close friends were HIV-positive. Many had close friends or family members who died of AIDS, often with little or no support from families, community institutions, social service agencies, and other organizations. The extent to which AIDS has affected people connected to LGBT communities cannot be overemphasized. The experience of Phil, an African American gay man, was all too typical, particularly for black gay men in the 1980s and 1990s. During his interview, Phil explained that in 1981 he had a dinner party with ten gay friends—all in their twenties and thirties. By 1991, all but two had died of AIDS. In ACT UP/Chicago and other chapters across the country, the grief and frustration involved in caring for sick comrades and attending far too many funerals contributed to a sense of rage and urgency.

For some interview respondents, one factor or the other played a decidedly primary role. Donald, an African American gay man in ACT UP/Chicago, was involved in leftist and anarchist politics prior to AIDS activism. He decided to get involved for "political reasons," viewing AIDS as a "genocidal attack against queers and people of color, and later I realized it was also an attack against women and the poor." He had little personal contact with HIV/AIDS until he became involved in the AIDS movement. Ellen, a bisexual white woman working at LA Shanti, was involved in the antiapartheid movement, the sanctuary movement (for Central American refugees), and others. As a bisexual, she gravitated politically toward fighting homophobia, and her work at a gay and lesbian center "naturally led to AIDS." In turn, her experience doing Latin American solidarity work led to a focus on AIDS in the Latino/a community. In contrast, Les, a black gay man in the U.S. military living in Los Angeles, had little activist experience prior to AIDS. His decision to take action was based on the large number of his civilian friends who were "dying from ignorance and denial."

For the majority of the respondents, the personal and the political dovetailed. Frank, a white gay activist in Los Angeles, was active in the Civil Rights movement, the antiwar movement, the student movement, the gay liberation movement and the Puerto Rican independence movement. This activist history, in tandem with seeing the devastation of AIDS and his own discovery that he was HIV-positive, led him to do AIDS work. Phil's comments reveal the intersection of personal

loss and his political consciousness as a black gay man: "I was los-
ing too many friends. . . . And I was angry because of what I saw. I
was just pissed. I would open *Newsweek* or *Time,* and any time I saw
HIV I saw white gay men. . . . It bore no resemblance to the reality
that I knew."

Virtually all the respondents reported that a key factor in the development of their political consciousness about AIDS was discrimination and prejudice targeting people with HIV/AIDS. When asked
about his motivations in becoming involved in AIDS activism,
Daniel, a gay white man in Chicago, stated: "I was pissed off at the
widespread ignorance and the widespread prejudice. That's why I became involved." Nearly all the respondents explicitly identified homophobia as a primary contributing factor in the spread of HIV/
AIDS and the lack of both compassion and services for PWA. In turn,
experiencing homophobia as gay men, lesbians, or bisexuals (or having a personal connection to the LGBT community) was also a significant factor in getting involved in AIDS activism.[2]

Thus, the data indicate that both the immediate, destructive impact of AIDS and immersion in activist networks were key factors in
the development of a collective AIDS consciousness. These factors
were closely linked to the social location of people affected by AIDS
(gays, lesbians, and bisexuals; people of color; women, etc.). Although there was a basic level of shared oppositional AIDS consciousness among activists in the study, there were also significant
differences—reflecting both oppositional and hegemonic consciousnesses. In the next section, I analyze how prior activism, social location, and collective identity factored into the divergent ideological
frames among AIDS activists.

Partial Oppositional Consciousness

Morris writes that political consciousness is "orientated toward either
the maintenance or the overthrow of a given system of domination"
(Morris 1992: 360). Patricia Hill Collins writes that domination "operates not only by structuring power from the top down but by simultaneously annexing the power as energy of those on the bottom
for its own ends" (Collins 1990: 227–228). Multiple forms of hegemonic consciousness extend into both oppressed communities and
social movement organizations and reinforce inequality. When a
group or individual expresses one form of oppositional consciousness

while simultaneously espousing hegemonic consciousness, partial oppositional consciousness exists. Examples include sexism and homophobia in antiracist struggles and racism and classism in feminist struggles. Thus, social change is inhibited not only by dominant society but by attitudes and practices within oppressed groups. The concept of partial oppositional consciousness provides a tool for looking at how multiple inequalities affect collective action. In turn, challenges to partial oppositional consciousness provide further insight into how intersectionality shapes social movement dynamics, the topic of Chapter 3.

As discussed in Chapter 1, a great deal of AIDS activism has involved challenging the multiple forms of oppression that nourish the spread of the disease. Consistent with black feminist theory, this oppression emanates not only from the federal government, media, medical establishment, and other dominant social institutions but from within oppressed communities themselves (Collins 1990; Davis 1983; Smith 1983). In her study, Cohen writes: "My aims required that I examine not only the obvious acts of dominant actors and institutions which inhibited mobilization, but also the indigenous norms, attitudes, and practices that influenced the participation and mobilization of those concerned about AIDS in African-American communities" (Cohen 1999: ix).

My research reveals that patterns of racism in the gay community, homophobia in heterosexual communities of color, sexism in both, and other forms of hegemonic consciousness were major obstacles to effective AIDS prevention and intervention. The ways in which individuals and organizations framed the crisis—how they understood it—were key in shaping strategic priorities, sparking internal divisions as well as building alliances between groups. Fierce ideological battles over how to frame the crisis and how to fight it were waged not only between marginalized communities and dominant society but between and within those communities themselves.

Divergent Ideological Frames

Analysis of the data reveals that there was significant ideological conflict within the AIDS movement. The data reveal a continuum on which varying ideological frames are located, ranging from one-dimensional to multidimensional with respect to systems of inequality. At one end of the continuum, individuals framed the AIDS crisis as a singular epidemic intertwined with homophobia but not fundamentally connected to racism, sexism, and classism. On the other end of the continuum, people perceived AIDS as an epidemic intertwined with homophobia as well as sexism, racism, and classism.

Many of the women and people of color interviewed (as well as more radical white gay men) criticized the predominantly middle-class white gay male sector of the AIDS movement for failing to address how race, gender, and class oppression were intertwined with the AIDS crisis. In one of the few social movement analyses of AIDS activism, Nancy Stoller writes about ACT UP: "Matters such as prevention and the development of a political analysis and strategy to combat racism, poverty, or sexism in the provision of services have had lower priority" (Stoller 1998: 151). Frank, a white gay member of ACT UP/Chicago with a history of leftist organizing, commented on how some activists rationalized their narrow framing of AIDS: "Another ideology within ACT UP represented by people like Peter Staley [a prominent ACT UP/New York member] has basically been: 'We can't cure racism, sexism, and other ills of society in our lifetime, but maybe we can cure AIDS.'" This singular crisis perspective is a concrete example of partial oppositional consciousness and was voiced by a significant number of white gay male activists in my research. These activists held ideological stances that opposed homophobia and related institutional neglect within the context of the AIDS crisis; but their relative complacency (and outright hostility at times) toward issues of race, sex, and class reflected their positions of privilege in other systems of oppression.

In one instance, after an ACT UP/Chicago meeting, Lyle, a white gay man, expressed dismay that someone had urged people at the meeting to attend an upcoming pro-choice event. In a subsequent discussion, he went on to say that "sexism and racism have nothing to do with AIDS." This perspective was articulated in interviews, meetings, and informal discussions by a number of white gay male activists. They often contended that focusing on racism and sexism diluted the strength of both the AIDS movement and the gay rights movement. Most white gay men interviewed for the study did not go so far as to say that race and gender played no role in the epidemic. Several even mentioned them as factors in the spread of HIV/AIDS. However, those that mentioned race and gender were less likely than women or people of color to discuss concrete ways in which racial and gender inequality affected the crisis. For example, Angelo, a white gay man in Stop AIDS Chicago, knew that people of color suffered disproportionate infection rates but was not able to offer any explanations as to why that was the case.

In contrast, people of color and women (largely gay men, lesbians, and bisexuals) were much more likely to view AIDS as connected to *multiple* oppressions and to discuss specific manifestations of racism, sexism, and classism within the AIDS crisis. In turn, they articulated specific plans of action for combating AIDS among people of color and women. For example, three of the Asian American respondents pointed out how Asians were undoubtedly underrepresented in statistics on AIDS-related deaths because family doctors often failed to pronounce AIDS as the cause of death and because many Asian immigrants with AIDS returned to their homelands to die. Virtually every woman interviewed critiqued clinical definitions of AIDS that ignored AIDS-related opportunistic infections in women as well as the dearth of research on and services for women, particularly poor women and women of color.

Activists with this *multidimensional* AIDS consciousness were more likely to situate their analyses and strategies within a larger political vision. For example, Frank situated AIDS activism within the context of national health care:

> I am attempting to steer some of this energy toward the nationwide debate on universal health care, which I believe will be a central point in U.S. society solving the AIDS crisis because I think if a cure were found tomorrow it wouldn't make its way into the bodies of people who use LA County Hospital for probably five years.

I use the term *multidimensional oppositional consciousness* to refer to a collective consciousness that emphasizes the importance of challenging multiple, interlocking oppressions. Here, it is important to point out that the concept is better conceptualized as an ideological or strategic goal rather than a completely inclusive ideology or strategy. In other words, few, if any, groups will be able to be inclusive of *every* inequality. As pointed out in the Preface, movement organizations need focus, but they should be aware of how other issues and inequalities interact with that focus. My point is that some individuals and organizations are further along the continuum with respect to being mindful of the complexity and interactions of oppressions in our society and around the world. As discussed earlier, this ideological perspective is rooted in the analyses of feminists of color and lesbian feminists who recognize that they are marginalized by more than one system of domination.

AIDS activists with this more inclusive consciousness articulated the need to battle racism, sexism, classism, and homophobia (and other inequalities such as ableism) related to the epidemic. This perspective often included criticisms of the partial oppositional consciousness prevalent among middle- and upper-class white gay men. Several interview respondents pointed out that the AIDS crisis is a health care crisis linked to preexisting inequities within the health care system. As Phil stated: "White gay men had to discover that they were not inheritors of the earth as they thought they might be. They were entitled to good health care. They had [it] until this fucking shit came up. And the rest of us were like, 'So what's new?'" Maria, a heterosexual Puerto Rican activist in New York City, pointed out:

> My view was that ACT UP was projecting AIDS as the only major health care problem in the nation. But as a matter of fact there are more women and children dying from domestic violence in the United States than of AIDS. And there's more people in our community dying of heart diseases and malnutrition than are dying of AIDS.

Maria's comments reflect the more complex consciousness more often articulated by women and people of color (again, disproportionately lesbians and gay men) in the AIDS movement. However, she presents a monolithic picture of ACT UP, a picture that ignores more progressive and radical ACT UP members. Interviews, discussions, and my own participant observation indicated that the radical ACT UP members believed that it *was* important to focus on AIDS (versus other issues) because societal responses to AIDS revealed how homophobia, racism, sexism, and classism permeated the government, medical establishment, media, and so on—and with such dire consequences for queers, people of color, and poor people.[3] Kate, a white heterosexual in ACT UP/Chicago, stated: "I can't say that AIDS is the *most* important issue and that's why I'm working on it. It's one issue that connects with all these other issues."

Within the AIDS movement, there were fierce debates about divergent framings of AIDS. In several cities, ACT UP chapters split over issues of race, class, and gender. Typically, one faction argued that race, class, and gender should not be central issues—"fighting AIDS" was the priority. The other faction typically argued that organizations cannot fight AIDS without combating the ways racism, sexism, classism, and homophobia were exacerbating the epidemic. In general, the former camp was composed of middle-class white gay men, frequently people living with HIV/AIDS. More often than not, these activists had little or no prior experience in social protest. The most blatant societal attack against them came in the form of AIDS and homophobia. Women (primarily lesbians) and people of color (mostly lesbians and gay men), as well as a small fraction of white gay men, formed the other group. This second group is also characterized by having prior activist experience.

Outside ACT UP, there were conflicts between predominantly white mega-agencies (Gay Men's Health Crisis in New York City and the AIDS Project Los Angeles) and smaller organizations in communities of color (to be discussed shortly). In turn, as mega-agencies were forced to take steps to be more inclusive, there was resentment from some white gay men. Mariko, a heterosexual Asian American woman, reported that AIDS Project Los Angeles was seen by many as an organization started by white gay men to serve white gay men and that as it shifted some of its resources to serve other communities (people of color, women), many white gay men reported feeling "abandoned" and "angry" and criticized the organization for straying from its original mission.

It is important to point out that the above analysis is somewhat oversimplified in two ways. First, hegemonic consciousness exists in virtually all oppressed communities. Emphasis has been placed on hegemonic racial and gender consciousness among middle- and upper-class white gay men in large part because they were among the first to engage in collective action to combat AIDS. The disproportionate impact on gay male communities and the conceptualization of AIDS as a "gay disease" logically resulted in gay communities being at the forefront of the movement.[4] Thus, other segments of the movement that developed later responded to existing organizations, which were disproportionately run by affluent white gay men. Hegemonic consciousness has also thwarted the AIDS movement within other communities, as is discussed in the next sections.

Second, the correlation between a person's social position and his or her political consciousness is by no means perfect. Although the data indicate that men are less likely to articulate an ideology and strategy that incorporates gender and whites are less likely to focus on race, oppositional consciousness is not an automatic result of social location. For example, some people of color contended that fighting racism should not be a priority in the fight against AIDS. The late Danny Sotomayor, a gay Latino AIDS activist, consistently argued that racism should not be a central priority for ACT UP/ Chicago.

In turn, there were white gay men—particularly those politically active prior to the AIDS epidemic—who displayed multidimensional oppositional consciousness. One clear example is Frank, an activist whose organizing has spanned four decades and various movements.

He pointed out that fighting AIDS in Los Angeles encompassed deal-ing with the aftermath of the Rodney King beating and the "underly-ing desperate social inequalities that exist on the basis of race and nationality here in LA. . . . The way in which the U.S. has dealt with the AIDS epidemic is only a symptom of much, much larger social problems in this country." Finally, although some continued to man-ifest partial oppositional consciousness, some white gay men (and others) developed a more inclusive oppositional consciousness. Frank noted: "There are a lot of white gay guys who have been moved toward a much more serious kind of progressive, antiracist, pro-women stance in relationship to the AIDS epidemic." In my own participation in ACT UP/Chicago, I observed white gay men, who had not been activists prior to AIDS, developing a more inclusive analysis of AIDS and other political issues and taking action in other areas, such as affordable housing for PWA.

Together, prior political experience and social location predicted ideology. The AIDS crisis exposed white gay men to the vagaries of the current health care system, sometimes catalyzing a militant, con-frontational response. However, lacking the social position or politi-cal experience or both, many failed to develop a more inclusive op-positional consciousness. In contrast, many activists with a history in progressive politics and antiracist or feminist ideologies—especially people of color and women—formulated a more complex framing of AIDS. Ideological tension related to political consciousness was evident within oppressed communities hit hard by AIDS and within AIDS organizations. The next sections provide greater detail on how partial oppositional consciousness affected the AIDS movement.

Sexism

Interview respondents stated that battling sexism in both communi-ties of color and gay male communities was central to AIDS organ-izing. Marion, an Afro-Caribbean heterosexual woman working with the Caribbean Women's Health Association in Brooklyn, stated that a central aspect of her agency's work involved challenging the "sub-servient roles" ascribed to women. For example, sexism translates into interactions that place women at risk for HIV, such as the refusal of many men (of all races) to wear condoms. Jan, an African Ameri-can lesbian, stated that the refusal of many men to wear condoms and the reluctance of women to demand them was a serious problem. She stressed the need for substantial education on "how we [women] view ourselves and our bodies in relation to men and how men view themselves also in terms of health and everything else."

Just as patriarchal consciousness led men to downplay the importance of gender oppression in the Civil Rights movement and the New Left (McAdam 1988; Echols 1989; Davis 1983), many gay male AIDS activists have failed to pay attention to the impact of AIDS on women (Corea 1992). Interviews and discussions with women in ACT UP as well as community-based AIDS agencies indicated that gay men often resisted including issues relating to women and AIDS as priorities. Decrying the lack of money for women's programs as "sexist," Yvonne, a black lesbian member of the AIDS Prevention Team in Los Angeles, asked, "Why is it that women don't count? And lesbians have been there for our gay brothers the whole time." Several lesbians stated that gay men resented the prominence of lesbians in the AIDS movement. Lesbians often came to ACT UP and other groups with more political organizing experience and played central leadership roles, and a number of gay men with whom I spoke felt threatened by female leadership. Tom, a white gay man in ACT UP/Chicago, accused lesbians of "dominating" the movement, going so far as to exclaim, "It was *our* movement first."

According to several men and women in New York City's Black AIDS Mobilization (BAM!), whose membership was composed primarily of black lesbians and gay men, sexism within the group was a problem. According to Ken, an African American gay man in BAM!, "I thought a lot of the men in the group were threatened by that fact [that the majority of members were lesbians]. A few of them were very misogynistic toward some of the women in the group." Ken remarked that some of the black gay men who were initially in the group left because they "could not handle" being in a group led by women.

Several women interviewed reported that men sometimes tried to ignore them during meetings and downplay the importance of HIV/AIDS initiatives targeting women. Ellen recalled a very important meeting she attended with the female assistant director of her agency. Ellen asserted that the male representative from the other organization, AIDS Project Los Angeles, was very sexist: "He didn't look at us straight in the eye once, didn't acknowledge our existence, only looked at and addressed the men in the room." Ellen felt slighted and angry, stating, "How can we work together if he won't even look at us?" It was one of the "worst meetings" she had ever been in, and nothing was accomplished. Kate related problems dealing with Ryan and Bobby, two white gay men in ACT UP/Chicago: "It's been a whole other area where I've had to kind of prove myself as being intelligent. And then the whole way the dynamics of conversation run—it's whoever screams the loudest or pushes their issue the most. . . . I feel like they're attacking me personally as well as attacking my ideas which just makes me totally shut down."

Other criticisms focused on the lack of attention to the ways in which AIDS affects women. Reflecting on the paucity of research and services targeting women affected by HIV/AIDS, Maria noted that when she began working at an AIDS clinic in the Bronx, there was no information on women and AIDS—"not even a flip chart on anatomy." In another instance, Gary, a white gay man in Chicago, complained about lesbian activists' calls for research on HIV risks for lesbian and bisexual women, stating that he saw no need for such research.

Nevertheless, my data also indicate that a significant number of gay men did perceive women's issues as important and worked in coalition with women's organizations. Although some men in BAM! did not stay with the group, a significant number remained. A majority of the gay men of color interviewed talked about the need to address the effect of AIDS on women, and several referred me to women who were active in the movement. More research is needed to examine what factors predict sensitivity on gender issues and if there are any differences in gender consciousness between gay men of color, white gay men, heterosexual men of color, and so on.

Racism

My interviews and participant observation suggest that hegemonic racial consciousness within gay male communities was an obstacle to AIDS prevention and intervention efforts targeting gay men of color. Prejudice, stereotypes, and exclusion have often served to either render gay men of color invisible or relegate them to marginal positions in relation to white gay male communities and organizations.

One representative example that illustrates the ways in which power dynamics within oppressed communities operate was described by two gay men (one Filipino, the other Filipino and black), working for the Asian Pacific AIDS Intervention Team in Los Angeles. While distributing condoms and safer sex literature in West Hollywood (a primarily white, middle- to upper-class gay area), they discovered a troubling dynamic in some gay interracial couples (Asian American men with white men). When outreach workers gave condoms and literature to an Asian American man, he often immediately gave them to his white partner. On some occasions, the white man returned the condoms to the outreach workers, stating, "He doesn't need these." The interview respondents linked such events to the subservient roles some Asian men play in interracial relationships with white men—relationships in which the white partner is the primary decisionmaker. Paralleling the effects of sexism in communities of color, racism in the gay community has impacts on interpersonal relationships.[5]

Paralleling black feminist criticisms of the mainstream women's movement (Davis 1983; Lorde 1984), black gay writer and activist Essex Hemphill (1991) noted that racism in the white gay community produced a predominantly white AIDS movement that was slow to deal constructively with the realities of people of color (see also Julien and Mercer 1991; Dalton 1991). Steven, a black gay ACT UP/Los Angeles member, stated: "White [AIDS] organizations are still basically dealing with AIDS even in 1993 as a white male queer disease." Interview respondents presented several interrelated criticisms of predominantly white, mainstream AIDS agencies. Particularly during the early years of the epidemic, the mega-agencies were typically staffed primarily by whites. During the late 1980s and early 1990s, some agencies put token people of color on staff and boards of directors rather than genuinely addressing racism in the organization—a dynamic that several respondents found repugnant.

Stephanie, an African American lesbian, recounted one incident involving tokenism and its effects on her. She was one of five ACT UP media coordinators for the Sixth International AIDS Conference in 1990. Stephanie stated that the media team consisted of "four white boys and me, which meant they could switch off, but I couldn't go anywhere because I was the only woman and the only person of color and I vowed never, ever to let that happen to me again because I couldn't go anywhere. I was always stuck because without me diversity went to hell." Stephanie was resentful about this and other similar incidents when she was the token black or female representative: "I learned very quickly not to allow myself to be used as an illusion of diversity."

Interview respondents linked underrepresentation of people of color in AIDS organizations to the issue of cultural insensitivity. Perhaps the most common example given is the failure to provide information and services in languages other than English. Other reported forms of cultural insensitivity included not having traditional foods at food banks and organizational events (such as Wonder Bread rather than tortillas for Latino/a immigrants in Los Angeles). Several respondents also stated that organizations and events were frequently located in places that were alienating to or inaccessible for many people of color (West Hollywood in Los Angeles, SoHo in New York City). Mike, a black gay man, commented on going to ACT UP/Los Angeles meetings: "There's something about driving into West Hollywood for a meeting that just turns people of color off because West Hollywood is so insidious in their own racism, in the gay racism. . . . It wasn't really centrally located. A lot of things they did seemed to perpetuate this old boy's club." These and other problems stemming from white racial insensitivity and ignorance made it more alienating for people of color to be active in many AIDS groups and more difficult for people of color to access AIDS-related services.

Interview respondents also criticized many white activists for not seeing how AIDS is linked to racial and class oppression and related social issues such as immigration, housing, and substance abuse. For example, Omar, a gay Latino activist in Los Angeles, mentioned that undocumented immigrants from Latin America were sometimes reluctant to get tested for HIV and seek out other services for fear of deportation. However, mainstream AIDS agencies often failed to provide immigrant-specific legal services to address such issues. Such services are particularly critical in areas such as California, where a strong wave of anti-immigrant hysteria persisted throughout the 1990s and continues today.

In some ACT UP chapters, there was considerable conflict between people of color caucuses and factions of the larger ACT UP body. Typically, people of color caucuses were set up to address the AIDS epidemic in communities of color. However, in many ACT UP chapters, when issues of race and AIDS were raised, there were members (primarily, but not exclusively, white gay men) who stated that fighting racism should not be a priority of the organization. One organization, Black AIDS Mobilization, was initially a caucus of ACT UP/New York but left after considerable conflict around racial issues (specifically about the larger group's lack of support for outreach in communities of color). Respondents from other cities related other problems, such as excessive scrutiny of spending by people of color caucuses and doubts expressed by white members about the ability of people of color to adequately articulate group demands at public events.[6] For example, when it was suggested that ACT UP/Chicago ask a representative of a Haitian organization to speak at a rally about the imprisonment of Haitians with HIV at Guantanamo Bay in 1993, Lyle, a white gay man, condescendingly stated that it would be difficult to find a Haitian who could deliver a speech that would "cover all the important points of the issue."

These dynamics were often accompanied by defensiveness among some whites, especially white men, and consequently anger among people of color. Steven reported that when he initiated a discussion on racism at an ACT UP/Los Angeles meeting, he and others were met with objections from white men, causing Steven to angrily state: "This is the crux of the problem. You're not listening. You're too busy being defensive. Just shut the fuck up and listen." Respondents in all three cities (New York, Los Angeles, and Chicago) stated that defensiveness around issues of race and racism among some white activists hindered the effectiveness of collective action.

Within ACT UP, white lesbians were far more likely to express concerns about racism and in general have been more active in AIDS issues that relate to people of color. This is not to say that white lesbians are immune to racial bias. However, evidence suggests that the prevalence of feminism and other progressive ideologies in the lesbian community plays a role in creating antiracist consciousness among white lesbians—a consciousness that is more rare among gay white men. Indeed, the radical feminist movement, although certainly troubled by its own racism, stimulated rigorous discussions on racism among white feminists, many of them lesbians (Taylor 1989; Echols 1989; Bulkin, Pratt, and Smith 1988)—something that has not happened on the same scale in gay male social movements. More research is needed on the interactions between feminist consciousness and antiracist consciousness.

Homophobia

Activists working in communities of color stated that AIDS activism has been hindered by apathy, denial, and intolerance rooted in homophobic consciousness. Many African American, Asian American, and Latino/a leaders have articulated the same homophobic messages as heterosexual, white male public officials, media spokespersons, and religious leaders.[7] Already lacking accessible health care and other resources, gay men of color have sometimes lost the support of their families and communities when they have needed it the most (Harris 1986; Dalton 1991; see essays in Hemphill 1991). Within the context of the AIDS epidemic, homophobia in communities of color serves to isolate not only gay men but other people with HIV and AIDS. According to Catalina,

> [Latino/a] family members often have many negative stereotypes of gay men. . . . Some of the gay men with HIV that I work with have been banished by their own families. It's almost like they believe these gay men deserve to get infected because of their "lifestyles." Many Latino families keep it [HIV/AIDS] hush-hush. There is one mother I work with that tells her children that she has cancer rather than AIDS.

According to most respondents, cultural taboos on sexuality, particularly homosexuality, have been at the core of resistance to explicit, public messages about AIDS prevention. As is the case in many white churches, many Christian churches (as well as Muslim mosques) in Asian American, African American, and Latino/a communities preach that homosexuality is a sin. Because AIDS is often perceived as a "gay disease" (and, indeed, effective AIDS prevention necessitates talking about homosexuality), these churches were often resistant to openly discussing it. As a result, churches, as well as other institutions and agencies, ignored transmission not only via homosexual sex but via heterosexual sex and sharing needles—thereby contributing to the ignorance and stigma that continue to fuel the spread of HIV/AIDS.

Most of the respondents of color reported that homophobia in the black, Latino/a, and Asian American communities made coalition building difficult. Churches frequently played a central role in the social life of these communities, but, according to respondents, churches in general resisted taking concrete actions to combat AIDS. As a consequence, challenging homophobia in churches has been a prerequisite to AIDS education. Yvonne, a black lesbian minister, commented that people often ignore

> the fact that there are gays and lesbians in their church who are African American, who have AIDS or who are HIV positive, who are afraid to come out of the closet because of the church's attitude on homosexuality. So I believe that we need to address homosexuality and religion . . . in order to help people to become more real about addressing AIDS in their own congregation or in their community.

Marco, a gay Latino activist, described a situation in which a nun who ran an "art space" in heavily Latino/a East Los Angeles refused to let Teatro Viva (a group of Latino/a queer artists) perform an educational theater piece on HIV/AIDS. According to Marco, the nun represented many middle-class, homophobic Latino/a homeowners in the area who viewed homosexuality as "immoral." In this and other similar instances, homophobia was an obstacle to educating communities of color about HIV/AIDS.

Homophobia is not only a problem in churches but in a vast array of community institutions. Activists stated that the reluctance of other institutions (including organizations such as the NAACP and the Urban League) to become active in the battle against AIDS has been due in large part to homophobia. In the early 1990s, Donald attempted to get Operation PUSH (a black community organization founded by Reverend Jesse Jackson, Sr.) to run an advertisement for a conference on AIDS in communities of color cosponsored by ACTUP/Chicago. According to Donald, PUSH refused to support the conference, stating that such a "pro–sexual liberation" stance was "not appropriate" for the black community. This situation relates to Cathy Cohen's finding that mainstream black leaders have sought to police the perceived "deviant" sexuality (including homosexuality) of community members in response to white society's historical use of negative images of black sexuality to perpetuate and justify racism.[8]

Classism

Although all the interview respondents were located within subordinate racial, sexual, and gender groups (there were no heterosexual white men among the interviewees), they tended to be privileged socioeconomically. There were several working-class and poor activists, but the majority of those I interviewed were middle class and college-educated (professionals, graduate students, human services workers). On the one hand, people of color interviewed were more likely to talk explicitly about class issues than whites, perhaps reflecting their own working class roots and/or more substantial interaction with working-class relatives and friends.[9] On the other hand, several of these respondents stated that class divisions often created tensions within communities of color. Being middle class tended to limit their interaction with poor and working-class people, inhibiting outreach and the formation of alliances. According to Ken, the running joke in BAM! was that you needed a college degree to be in the group. He stated that the middle-class, professional status of most of the group made it difficult for them to gain entree into working-class black communities. Patricia, a black bisexual in BAM!, concurred: "And certainly those people [poor or working-class African Americans] wouldn't have stayed around long. I just don't feel like we were as sensitive to that as we should have been—or even could have been."

Kyle, a black gay activist in New York City, stated that "lesbian and gay activism and even AIDS activism to a degree is a privilege in this society, and I think you have to have a certain status in order to do it." Certainly, there are poor and working-class gay and lesbian activists, but Kyle's comments are instructive. He stressed the importance of being mindful of class privilege, particularly within the context of direct action protest involving the possibility of arrest. The costs of being arrested (aside from the increased likelihood of people of color being brutalized by the police) include raising bail money and missing work—both of which weigh more heavily on working-class and poor people (to be discussed further in Chapter 5).

Several activists of color criticized both grassroots organizations in communities of color and ACT UP for lacking a class analysis. Steven, an ACT UP/Los Angeles member, labeled a community-based black gay AIDS group as "bourgeois," criticizing the organization for not being more confrontational tactically. Although Steven's critique may be conflated with a conflict of opinion over tactics, his critique was echoed by other activists, who criticized AIDS service agencies for using funding for high salaries and plush office spaces rather than expanding services and programs for poor and working-class clients. In addition, there was sometimes resentment among direct action activists that mainstream agencies received funding (e.g., Ryan White Care Act monies) that was the product of years of confrontational grassroots protest.

One emblematic case of class conflict was reported by former members of the Latino Caucus of ACT UP/New York. This conflict, which contributed to the disbanding of the caucus, involved a campaign to challenge the Hispanic AIDS Forum (HAF)—an organization whose stated goal was to provide services to people, particularly Latinos/as, affected by HIV/AIDS in New York City. Interview respondents Javier and Carlos, both in ACT UP/New York's Latino Caucus, stated that HAF was located in SoHo—an area in southern Manhattan that was "worlds away" from the majority of the Latino/a population of New York in Harlem, Brooklyn, and the Bronx. They also reported that the agency did not have any openly gay or HIV-positive people on its board of directors and thus did not represent people living with HIV/AIDS. Finally, they criticized HAF for failing to make any substantive attempts to do outreach in the Latino/a community and failing to set up programs for which it had received government funding.

Javier and Carlos stated that when members of the Latino Caucus proposed a plan to publicly challenge HAF's inaction, other caucus members opposed the idea because it involved attacking a Latino/a organization. The interview respondents, however, felt that the core issue was class, not "racial solidarity." They stated that opposing members of the caucus (as well as the agency itself) were using race as an excuse not to deal with their own class privilege. HAF members reportedly complained that ACT UP used a model that was "alien" to the Latino/a community, claiming that the Latino/a community did not understand marching, chanting in the streets, and so on. However, Javier, Carlos, and other Latino Caucus members felt that HAF staff members were disconnected from the Latino/a community, being primarily politically conservative, upper middle class, and heterosexual. Javier labeled this contradiction as a "conflict of political ideology" and asserted that in contrast to HAF's perspective, social change in Latino/a communities came through street activism, direct action, strikes, sit-ins, violence, and other forms of activism. He felt that the administrators and board at HAF were using this racial argument to protect their lucrative positions in the AIDS bureaucracy.

In a similar situation, Elena, a bisexual Puerto Rican working with the alternative AIDS clinic VIDA/SIDA, critiqued Chicago's Hispanic AIDS Network for acquiring $1 million in funding: "They've never done anything that I know of that's been helpful to the community. . . . They're opportunistic. . . . The only ones that benefited were the ones with big positions in it. They used people with AIDS." This dynamic is key to understanding the sociology and politics of HIV/AIDS in the twenty-first century, when AIDS has become a veritable "industry," in which chief executive officers of pharmaceutical companies make millions yearly and AIDS agency directors make six-digit salaries, while those living in poverty comprise a highly disproportionate number of those living with HIV/AIDS.

Interview respondents tended to focus commentary on class dynamics within communities of color, but at least two activists criticized the failure of many AIDS activists to recognize the marginalized position of working-class and poor white people within the AIDS crisis. In one instance, Donald criticized other members of ACT UP for wanting to restrict a conference agenda to people of color and to not include working-class or poor white people. Stephanie stated that people are always ready to include black and Latina women in discussions on women and AIDS but tend to gloss over the severe impact of AIDS on poor white women.[10]

When Consciousnesses Clash:
Contested Definitions and Controversial Analogies

Collective action is complicated by competing definitions of what constitutes both hegemonic and oppositional consciousness. Actions may be framed within the context of one stream of consciousness by one activist and in a quite different way by another. The Hispanic AIDS Forum's political positions were labeled as classist by some members of the Latino Caucus but were seen as maintaining racial solidarity in the Latino/a community in the face of the white-dominated AIDS movement by others.

Another example concerns opposition to clean needle exchanges in communities of color. Some black and Latino/a leaders have condemned such programs, claiming that they promote drug addiction and therefore contribute to racial genocide. It is at times difficult to disentangle this argument, which is certainly seen by its proponents as a form of racial oppositional consciousness (i.e., "zero tolerance for drugs in communities of color"), from the widespread prejudice targeting injection drug users that is promoted by the criminalization of addiction. In my research, many AIDS activists perceived the criminalization of addiction as part and parcel of the racism and classism embedded in the criminal justice system. Throughout the 1980s and 1990s, injection drug users composed a disproportionate number of those infected with HIV in the United States. They have faced hatred and scorn from the general public (including communities of color) and systemic neglect from the government. At a time when clean needle exchanges and rehabilitation programs were sorely needed, government funding was woefully inadequate, and increasing numbers of addicted, disproportionately poor people and people of color were thrown in prisons across the country. From this perspective, advocacy for clean needle exchanges is rooted in oppositional consciousness challenging the racist and classist war on drugs (see Lusane 1991; Patton 1990; Reiman 1995).

The merging of (hegemonic) heterosexist consciousness and (oppositional) racial consciousness often serves to equate gayness with being white and being "of color" with being heterosexual, particularly within the context of dominant perceptions of masculinity. In other words, people of color are seen as monolithically heterosexual, and lesbians and gay men are seen as monolithically white, which ignores the lives of millions of LGBTs of color. This compartmentalization of race and sexuality was (and continues to be) articulated in the mainstream media and other dominant institutions. This reporting on a shift in HIV infection from the "gay community" to "communities of color" during the late 1990s often negated the existence of gay men of color and their high rates of HIV/AIDS since the beginning of the epidemic. Unfortunately, even progressive news media perpetuate the false dichotomy of race and sexuality. In an article in *Mother Jones*, a progressive magazine, Jacob Levenson (2000) examines the impact of HIV/AIDS in the black community but fails to discuss or even acknowledge black gay and bisexual men, who continue to be the group hardest hit by the epidemic.

Several activists reported that members of communities of color often believe that being gay or lesbian and being of color are mutually exclusive. Yvonne described an incident that typifies this dichotomous and destructive political consciousness. She began by quoting the secretary at a black church in Los Angeles with whom she had spoken:

> "Gays and lesbians deserve every right that any other person has. . . ." She [the secretary] was so emphatic, and I was so proud. I thought, "Wow—what consciousness. I didn't even realize that there was that much positive out there. . . ." She said, "They deserve every right as African Americans." And I said, "Yes, the African American gays and lesbians deserve every right as anybody else." And there was complete silence. I broke her. . . . I caught the fact that she was saying gays and lesbians, but she was talking about white people . . . and not willing to acknowledge that there are African American gays and lesbians in her own church.

Jack, an African American gay man, recounted an experience he had while talking with Charlene, another AIDS activist, at an AIDS conference. Upon learning that Jack was gay, Charlene, a black heterosexual woman, said, "You people have been at the table too long. It's time to let black people come to the table and talk about the services that are needed in the black community. And I'm like lookin' at her like 'Hello. Look, I'm black too.' And I told her that was really insulting." Such interactions were reported by other African American, Asian American, and Latino/a interview respondents. Charlene's comments illustrate how hegemonic (heterosexual) consciousness and oppositional (black) consciousness can coexist in one individual. This consciousness, which equates being gay with being white, makes it extremely difficult for lesbians and gay men of color to merge racial and sexual identities in a racist, homophobic society (see Anzaldúa 1987; Navarro 1991; Hemphill 1991; Beam 1986; Lorde 1982). Jack stated that this mindset is common and that he has had to inform people that being a gay man "doesn't mean I don't identify with being black."[11]

Some people see heterosexist consciousness as consistent with black, Asian, or Latino/a "militancy" or "tradition." In denigrating gay men and lesbians, whom they see as assimilated into dominant white culture, they also alienate a segment of their own community—lesbians and gay men of color. According to interview respondents, this is one factor that isolates many gay men of color and prevents them from seeking out AIDS-related services. In turn, homophobia forces many gay and bisexual men to stay in the closet and sometimes to have unprotected sex with women. The marginalization of lesbians and gay men in communities of color is particularly disturbing, given the tremendous contributions to the fight against AIDS made by many gay men and lesbians of color, such as the late filmmaker and activist Marlon Riggs. His films *Tongues Untied, No Regrets,* and *Black Is, Black Ain't* explore controversial issues related to race, sexuality, AIDS, and other issues. The ideological exclusion of LGBTs from communities of color illustrates the consequences of the intertwining of "antiracist" consciousness and homophobic consciousness and demonstrates the interactive character of different forms of political consciousness.[12]

An activist's collective consciousness also influences her or his conceptions of what constitutes "activism" and being an "activist." Verta Taylor and Nancy Whittier note that social movement participants engage in "negotiation" as they attempt to construct a collective identity: "Negotiation encompasses the symbols and everyday actions subordinate groups use to resist and restructure existing systems of domination" (Taylor and Whittier 1992: 111). The data indicate that the existence of multiple inequalities complicates the process of this negotiation, creating a situation in which activist symbols are contested. Within the AIDS movement, the "uniforms" of activism have become linked to certain brands of consciousness and activism. Mike, an ACT UP/Los Angeles member, linked the communication problems between ACT UP–style activists and mainstream AIDS activists to appearance, stating that he managed to

> get a core of volunteers who were young, radical, out-there faggots that were really wanting to do a good cause, but we were stopped because if you have Mr. Brooks Brothers AIDS activist coming into contact with an AIDS activist wearing Doc Martens [black combat boots] and has all these piercings and all these tattoos, there's no communication.

Here, Mike described the style of dress for many ACT UP members, a uniform that is intertwined with one form of collective *queer* identity. This uniform presents a challenge not only to dominant heterosexual society but also to mainstream, assimilationist gay men and lesbians. The situation is even more complex. Frank criticized some ACT UP activists' narrow vision of activism, again linking fashion and consciousness:

> It's always been difficult to persuade ACT UP types, in particular, that in communities of color there are AIDS activists because ACT UP doesn't see any people with black combat boots and earrings in communities of color so it's their assumption that there are no AIDS activists, and they tend, therefore, to dismiss AIDS service organizations that exist in those communities that are activist in just as serious a way as they are and, in effect, frequently more serious but less noisy.

Thus, Frank perceived a shortsightedness on the part of those ACT UP members who displayed a queer oppositional consciousness but failed to recognize that their style of political action may not be the only progressive or militant one, particularly within communities of color.

Another movement dynamic that illustrates the complexity of multiple political consciousnesses was evidenced in the resentment that some of the interview respondents, primarily African Americans, harbored toward analogies made between the Civil Rights movement and the gay and lesbian movement (Civil Rights legislation, gay marriage). Tabitha, a black lesbian, emphasized that many white lesbians and gay men doing "consciousness raising" about lesbian and gay rights in communities of color failed to realize that individuals' experiences as people of color affect how they perceive messages coming from a white lesbian or gay man. White gay and lesbian communities have seldom expressed solidarity with communities of color, and when they come to communities of color for solidarity, in Tabitha's words, "it rings hollow." In Tabitha's mind, this mistrust is exacerbated by parallels made between homophobia and racism as well as between the LGBT movement and the Civil Rights movement: "They [white lesbians and gay men] could never understand why black people would just explode whenever they brought the analogy up."

There is no doubt that the anger many black heterosexuals feel about comparisons between "black" and "gay" movements is frequently motivated by homophobia (and accompanying ignorance of homophobic oppression and LGBT political struggles). Indeed, many heterosexuals (black and nonblack) do not view homophobia as a form of oppression; rather, they see homosexuality as morally wrong. However, the strong reaction of many African American lesbians and gay men reflects a more attentive analysis of history and contemporary politics. Like Tabitha, many black lesbians and gay men feel that it is hypocritical for white gay men and lesbians to use images of black political struggle to advance their own cause while simultaneously perpetuating racism within gay and lesbian communities. In the words of Julien and Mercer: "Although gays derived inspiration from the symbols of Black liberation, they failed to return the symbolic debt, by proceeding to ignore racism" (Julien and Mercer 1991: 168). Other gay and lesbian people of color also resented analogies made between antiracist and gay and lesbian struggles. Noel, a Filipino gay man, stated that

> the self-appointed white lesbian and gay leaders were talking about people of color. I started getting furious because they started making analogies to the 1960s black Civil Rights movement, and I thought how dare they when it's not the same movement, and they started to create gay as another racial minority and it's just, "no girl, we [people of color] gotta do our own party."

Noel's comments indicate that he sees a clear connection between antiblack and anti-Asian racism and between the Civil Rights movement and Asian American–Pacific Islander movements. This again raises the issue of the central role that black political struggles have played in relation to political struggles in other communities.[13]

Multiple Sites of Oppression

On a broad level, the "problem" of AIDS exemplifies the different sites of power and oppression in U.S. society. Not only is domination clearly linked to an oppressive political regime (whether it be Reagan, George H. W. Bush, Clinton, or George W. Bush) and a capitalist economic system that values profits over human lives, but also power operates through other myriad institutions, networks, and cultural beliefs—on the community and interpersonal levels. Clearly, as seen in this chapter, multiple consciousnesses and interlocking oppressions operating within communities of color and gay and lesbian communities impeded efforts to build a more inclusive, effective AIDS movement.

The data provide an opportunity to build upon the growing body of literature examining how multiple systems of human domination affect collective consciousness and action (Morris 1992; Collins 1990; Davis 1983). Vincent Roscigno writes: "When examining group struggle, it is also crucial to recognize the interactive nature of inequality processes and the embeddedness of such processes in social organization. Indeed, these considerations can have a substantial impact upon the extent to which insurgency has its desired result" (Roscigno 1994: 118). The data also support the black feminist tenet (Combahee River Collective 1983) that multiple systems of oppression are interlocking. The AIDS crisis cannot be understood by looking at different forms of inequality in isolation. Various communities are affected by multiple inequalities. As seen in the data, denial and apathy rooted in homophobia in communities of color have impeded prevention and intervention efforts as African Americans, Asian Americans, and Latinos/as continue to become infected with HIV. This homophobia must be analyzed within the context of racial oppression. The compartmentalization of race and sexuality (i.e., "gay" = "white") that is one facet of homophobia in communities of color represents a racialized response to homosexuality (i.e., homosexuality as another "white" threat to the racial community). An analysis of AIDS and homophobia in communities of color must take into account the ways in which racial oppression influences responses to homosexuality. For example, gay men of color have unique HIV/AIDS-related issues linked to their social location at the intersection of multiple oppressions. Intervention efforts must take into account not only how gay men of color are affected by racism, homophobia, and classism emanating from the dominant society but also how they are affected by the particular manifestations of both homophobia in communities of color and racism in LGBT communities.

Other forms of partial oppositional consciousness within communities struck by AIDS have also impeded collective action. Sexism—in communities of color and gay communities—often serves to silence the voices of women, thereby inhibiting the creation of strategies to combat AIDS among women. Racism within primarily white gay organizations contributes to the dissemination of prevention messages and services that are alienating and/or inaccessible for people of color. Class divisions in various communities serve to inhibit the formation of programs that address the complex needs of poor and working-class people within the context of the AIDS crisis. The disproportionately high rates of HIV infection among those at the intersections, particularly poor women of color and gay and bisexual men of color, reflect the interactive effects of different forms of oppression on the epidemic, effects that are compounded by partial oppositional consciousness.

The data suggest that partial oppositional consciousness can be conceptualized as one of the ideological bolts that hold together systems of domination. Patterns of oppression within oppressed communities operate to protect hegemonic consciousness and thus reinforce dominant social structures. In other words, those at the top of the power structure do not have to do as much work because people in marginalized communities sometimes engage in oppressive behavior themselves, leaving dominant groups unscathed and their privilege and power intact.[14]

Given the existence of multiple oppressions, Morris (1992) raises the issue of whether or not any system of domination is primary. Most of the people of color and white lesbians (and some of the gay white men) interviewed emphasized the necessity of fighting all forms of oppression. They critiqued activist approaches that prioritized one form of inequality because such approaches did not take into account the other inequalities that constrained their lives. Critiquing a narrow focus on gay rights, Phil provided the following image in which he, as a gay black man, comes to a door with a set of signs that says: "'No queers allowed. No blacks allowed. No women allowed.' No whatever. I could buy into your agenda and take the 'No queers allowed' sign off. I still could not get through that fucking door. And then you would get through that door, and you'd slam it shut."

Although fiercely committed to struggling against sexism, homophobia, and racism, several interview respondents stated that class oppression is a commonly overlooked stratifying force that inhibits consciousness and collective action. Jeff, an Asian American–Pacific Islander gay man in New York City, stated: "I think a lot of activists are closeted about class. . . . People's perspectives are rooted in their class background." Some activists viewed class consciousness as a core component of more radical, inclusive collective action frames that held promise for unifying different oppressed groups. For example, Javier concluded, "We have to be able to formulate some type of ideology on class. . . . Until that happens we won't be able to connect all the isms." This comment suggests that social movement scholars as well as activists might do well to follow the advice of Mayer Zald (1992) and Rick Fantasia (1989), who state that there is a need to more explicitly link class analysis to social movement theory. Because my sample was disproportionately middle class, it would be useful to interview more poor and working-class activists to analyze their experiences and ideologies.

Activists' comments about collective consciousness were not restricted to the areas of gender, race, sexuality, and class. Interview respondents involved in the Puerto Rican independence movement consistently placed AIDS and other social problems within the context of U.S. colonialism and neocolonialism. Maria asserted that AIDS is part of larger health care issues that relate to the "genocide" of Puerto Rican people: "As an oppressed nationality, as a colonized nation, we have a larger scale of issues that we have to work on. AIDS or housing or education are all a part of that agenda." Alberto, a Puerto Rican gay man, stated that the "question of AIDS in my community is a colonialist issue and because of that I'll struggle against it." Within the context of anticolonial political struggles, oppositional consciousness can also be "partial." For example, if "nationality" preempts sexuality, gender, race, or class, then the unique ways in which Puerto Rican queers, women, and poor people are affected by HIV/AIDS will not be confronted.

The AIDS crisis also suggests that new forms of collective consciousness and beliefs may emerge along with related social categories. Several respondents discussed AIDSphobia, a term that refers to the prejudice, discrimination, and other forms of inequality facing people with AIDS or HIV. Since the 1980s, there have been numerous efforts to codify the stigmatization of people living with HIV, including criminal transmission laws, mandatory reporting of the names of people living with HIV/AIDS, proposals for quarantine or expulsion, and so on. AIDS activists themselves have not been immune to AIDSphobia. Steven, an HIV-positive member of ACT UP/ Los Angeles, stated that a few HIV-negative, "HIVphobic" men in ACT UP would not room with HIV-positive members during out-of-town demonstrations and broke up with HIV-positive boyfriends. One BAM! member stated that people in the organization virtually never discussed the issue of HIV/AIDS within the group itself and thought that an HIV-positive person would probably feel uncomfortable being in the organization.

In turn, people with HIV and AIDS have constructed HIV/AIDS-positive oppositional consciousness that challenges the stigmatization and exclusion produced by AIDSphobia. This consciousness is expressed by being very open about being infected with HIV—speaking publicly about living with HIV/AIDS, wearing T-shirts and buttons indicating one's positive status, or even wearing a necklace with a vial of one's HIV-positive blood, as did one ACT UP member I knew. As someone diagnosed with HIV in 1995, I derived inspiration and support from those who had struggled for more than a decade before me.[15] The development of new oppositional identities calls attention to the need for a conceptual framework that analyzes multiple, evolving systems of oppression.

One finding that is clear is that various forms of community-level inequality often operate simultaneously. The data reveal situations in which individuals and organizations face the compounded effects of multiple spheres of domination. Activists are faced with multiple forms of hegemonic consciousness simultaneously. Black lesbians in BAM! argued with black gay men over gender issues and with white ACT UP members over race while also grappling with their own class privilege. Members of ACT UP/New York's Latino Caucus faced white paternalism in ACT UP, homophobia while organizing in the Latino/a community, and conflicts over class divisions within the caucus itself. Mariko, an Asian American activist, faced severe difficulties recruiting "buddies" for PWA in South Central Los Angeles in the early 1990s. Mariko stated that most black churches in the community were not interested in getting involved in AIDS work, and most of the volunteers were white and did not want to travel to South Central.

Victor's experiences as an African American, bisexual, HIV-positive prisoner vividly illustrate the confluence of different spheres of domination. As a black prisoner with HIV, Victor faced the compounded effects of race and class oppression related to incarceration (Stockdill 1995), as well as prejudice and discrimination from other inmates because of his sexuality and HIV status. He wrote various AIDS organizations—including the Kupona Network, a black AIDS organization in Chicago—virtually none of which even responded to his requests for information and support. It is significant, in this context, that a mostly white, middle-class organization—ACT UP/Chicago—*did* respond to Victor and support him. This support reflected the radical oppositional consciousness of ACT UP/Chicago's Prison Issues Committee, as will be discussed in Chapter 4.

Oppositional AIDS consciousness is predicted by activist history and being personally affected by AIDS. The breadth of this oppositional consciousness is also shaped by these factors. Those respondents previously immersed within activist networks, particularly people of color and women, were more likely to express a multidimensional oppositional consciousness than those whose first activist experience occurred in the AIDS movement, disproportionately (but not exclusively) middle-class white gay men. Within the AIDS crisis, activists identified various forms of partial oppositional consciousness as barriers to effective prevention and intervention work. This situation is further complicated by conflicting notions of oppositional consciousness and activism. Logically, strategies are affected by ideology and consciousness. The next two chapters focus on different strategies emanating from multidimensional oppositional consciousness.

3

Forging Unity:
Grassroots AIDS Activism
in Communities of Color

My role—if nothing else—is to remind people and ourselves that
AIDS is much more complex than we think . . . that PWAs can become people with disabilities, that PWAs come in all sizes and
shapes and colors etc., that sexism has everything to do with AIDS,
that discrimination has everything to do with AIDS, that health is
a control issue, and it's a power issue, it's a privilege issue.
    —Jeff, an Asian American–Pacific Islander gay AIDS activist

Jeff's words reflect an oppositional consciousness attentive to multiple
inequalities that was expressed in many of the interviews with AIDS activists of color—particularly lesbians, bisexuals, and gay men. For the
activists of color I interviewed, this multidimensional oppositional consciousness was translated into grassroots strategies that simultaneously
challenged racism, sexism, classism, and homophobia within the AIDS
crisis.

Social movement theories, however, tend to look at collective action that targets singular forms of oppression and thus do not capture
this world of activism. In an attempt to fill in this void, in this chapter I analyze multifaceted efforts to increase awareness about AIDS,
empower people in affected communities, and improve HIV/AIDS
programs and services. These community-level strategies represent
the crucial cultural and consciousness-raising work that is at the core
of much of progressive AIDS activism. Analyzing strategies directed

at promoting collective consciousness that challenges multiple inequalities on multiple levels—consciousness that optimally leads to
both individual and collective action—interjects the concept of intersectionality into current dialogues on collective action.

Mobilization Strategies

The organizations analyzed for this chapter were primarily community-based organizations in communities of color; many still exist
today. In general, they had two primary, immediate goals: to prevent
the spread of HIV transmission and to provide treatment, support,
and social services to people living with HIV and AIDS. Organizational efforts focused on the following areas: street-level prevention
efforts (distribution of condoms, dental dams,[1] and safer sex information); support services for people living with HIV (treatment issues, emotional support); assistance with related social problems (immigration, housing, health care, substance abuse, food); promotion of
positive images of lesbians and gay men, especially lesbians and gay
men of color; and efforts to shape public policy and public opinion
about HIV/AIDS through education and social protest.

As discussed in Chapter 2, many interview respondents saw AIDS
prevention and intervention as inseparable from challenging multiple
inequalities and related social problems such as poverty and the criminalization of addiction. In addition to challenging local, state, and
federal governments, the media, and the medical establishment, this
approach involved challenging inequalities on the community level
(i.e., partial oppositional consciousness). Mobilization strategies to
galvanize multidimensional oppositional consciousness and catalyze
both individual and collective action in the face of the AIDS crisis can
be placed in four interrelated categories: (1) constructive dialogue, (2)
empowerment initiatives, (3) community embeddedness, and (4) use
of cultural traditions.

Constructive Dialogue

Josh Gamson's (1989) research on AIDS activism demonstrates that
instrumental tactics (protesting a dominant institution's actions or in-
actions) and cultural or expressive tactics (publicly challenging prej-
udiced cultural beliefs) are not mutually exclusive. They may be used
separately or simultaneously, depending on the target of collective
action.[2] Within my study, respondents reported a range of strategies

and tactics that varied according to the target and goals (other factors included the potential for repression, which is discussed in Chapter 5). The locus of AIDS activism *within* communities of color and LGBT communities (as opposed to activism targeting dominant white and heterosexual culture and institutions) has been an important factor shaping the methods used to promote social change. Strategies to combat partial oppositional consciousness within oppressed communities and within the AIDS movement itself, by and large, differ from strategies to combat oppression directly linked to dominant institutions.

The interviews reveal the use of constructive dialogue as a central tactic to confront community-level inequality. Within the direct action group ACT UP, women's caucuses and people of color caucuses scheduled numerous in-house educational events designed to increase sensitivity and knowledge around gender and racial inequality. Steven, an African American gay man in ACT UP/Los Angeles, spoke on how people of color and women worked to challenge the perception that only affluent white gay men are affected by AIDS: "It's more than just doing the physical work—it's also the changing of consciousness. . . . You have to tell these white boys over and over, 'No, it's not your fucking disease.'" Although such internal discussions were sometimes quite heated, they reflect that activist's commitment to expand the oppositional consciousness of other ACT UP members. During the early 1990s, such internal education was key in expanding ACT UP chapters' campaigns to include housing, needle exchange, prison issues, and other areas.

Writing about responses to AIDS in black communities, Cathy Cohen states that "in contrast to the more aggressive political tactics of civil disobedience, the political strategies in African American communities were much less confrontational, with compromise and education being key" (Cohen 1999: 341). Stephanie, an African American lesbian in ACT UP/Chicago—an organization that engaged in extremely confrontational, militant tactics against the medical establishment and the government—advocated a different approach to dealing with black funeral parlor directors who were illegally overcharging the families of people who had died of AIDS. In this case, rather than organizing a demonstration, she and other AIDS activists sat down with the funeral directors and carefully explained that it would be better for all parties involved if the problem was solved through negotiation and without publicity. Although there was a clear message that "the shit would hit the fan" if they did not change their policy, Stephanie stressed that it was crucial to "let them [the funeral parlor directors] know you're coming at them with respect and brotherhood and sisterhood." Another example illustrates the use of dialogue within communities of color. New York City–based Black AIDS Mobilization used picketing and civil disobedience leading to arrests to protest the Immigration and Naturalization Service's racist and xenophobic imprisonment of Haitians with AIDS at the Guantanamo Bay military base. The same group performed educational outreach about homophobia and AIDS in African American communities and engaged in constructive criticism and internal discussions about sexism in the organization itself.

Challenging homophobia in communities of color often took place on a one-to-one basis or in workshops and presentations. One AIDS organization serving the Caribbean community in Brooklyn, New York, set up a home visitor program in which outreach workers went into people's homes to encourage dialogue around the taboo subjects of sex and sexuality. According to Marion, a heterosexual Afro-Caribbean woman, the results were "amazing," and a significant change occurred in many families' willingness to openly discuss topics related to HIV and AIDS. AIDS outreach programs created by other organizations reported similar successes. Activists linked this type of success to the fact that outreach workers were trained in the biology, psychology, and social aspects of AIDS and, most important, came from the targeted communities themselves.

Activist strategies differentiated between dominant social institutions and marginalized communities. In general, activists worked very hard to avoid public conflict when responding to inequities within their own communities. Although conflict did at times occur, activists more often attempted to facilitate dialogue about problematic issues to build alliances that could be utilized to fight not only AIDS but other social problems. Tactics were shaped by a strategy to build coalitions that rest upon existing cultures of resistance but also seek to expand this oppositional culture to include more than one form of oppositional consciousness.

Dialogue, however, is only one step toward fostering oppositional consciousness. Tabitha, a black lesbian, remarked that AIDS education goes deeper than telling people to use a condom: "You have to change people's ideas and the way they look at themselves and the way they perceive their bodies and their place in society; if people don't feel that they're that important to begin with, then 'oh what the hell.'" A key element in the transformation of collective consciousness involves empowerment. Particularly for poor people and other marginalized groups, reframing the situation as a collective injustice, an act of consciousness raising, must be accompanied by a change in the potential participant's sense of agency—on both an individual and collective level.

Empowerment Initiatives

One emphasis in current social movement scholarship involves conceptualizing the connections between individual and collective levels of mobilization. William Gamson (1992) presents the concept of "microevents"—events that link individual and cultural levels and, optimally, facilitate the mobilization of consciousness and action. The interviews suggest that, within the AIDS movement, successful microevents have been guided by a model of empowerment that pays attention to the complex social forces affecting people's lives.

Interview respondents reported that they spent a considerable amount of time developing strategies to facilitate individual empowerment. Through support groups, educational workshops, and one-on-one interactions, activists worked to educate and promote self-worth and dignity among people affected by HIV/AIDS. Many community-based service organizations set up mechanisms to involve clients in the organization—both in decisionmaking processes and helping other clients. Peer educators were key, as in the alternative AIDS clinic VIDA/SIDA's peer tutor program in Chicago, in which young people from the Latino/a community were trained in the science, psychology, and cultural issues of AIDS and then conducted a door-to-door educational campaign. According to Alberto and Elena, the peer educators were very well received in most homes and loved their jobs so much that they even continued to work after funding for the program was cut.

Stephanie noted that a primary aspect of her job at the Chicago Women's AIDS Project was to help develop a sense of "entitlement" among women with HIV and AIDS so that they were better able to demand housing, health care, and so on. In addition to helping people to see that they are entitled to a certain standard of living, activists emphasized the importance of dealing with various everyday problems in poor people's lives. Maria, a Puerto Rican activist, stated: "If you ask a woman with HIV, 'what are your problems?' she's not gonna tell you AIDS. She's gonna tell you, 'Well, I don't have a house to live in. I don't have food for all my children.'" While doing street outreach, Tabitha encountered a woman who said she did not want a condom because she had a drug problem and

when she's high, she doesn't care what she does and her life is so
fucked up anyway that she's dying, so what the hell does she care
if she gets HIV/AIDS? It's no worse than anything else she has to
live through. . . . She could just put it together in a way that a lot of
policymakers just can't see. That kind of connection is imperative.

Tabitha asserted that mobilizing people—whether for individual or
collective action—requires a holistic approach that deals with the
various social realities (e.g., homelessness, addiction, lack of child-
care, welfare and poverty, domestic violence) of marginalized communities: "It's got to be linked to providing services that the community needs in some real way." When people see that there is a
possible way to meet their basic needs, they are more likely to be
motivated to take action to change their lives (e.g., seek out health
care or drug rehabilitation) and, in turn, work with others on a collective level (e.g., become a peer educator). This dynamic was reported by several activists in community-based organizations, who
talked about (or were themselves) clients who later became activists.
Jackie, a bisexual Native American who identifies culturally as a
Latina, first became a client at the Chicago Women's AIDS Project
and then emerged as both a vocal client advocate for that group and
an outspoken ACT UP/Chicago activist living with AIDS.

Their awareness of the complex layers of systemic exclusion and
adversity that undergird the AIDS epidemic enabled these and other
activists to develop programs that were effective. According to Omar,
a gay Latino, Bienestar, a Latino AIDS program in Los Angeles, offered (and still offers) services that satisfied many of the needs of
community members. Services and information were provided in
English and Spanish. Information was available at the agency's drop-
in center and various other sites, such as community festivals and
day laborer's camps. The clinic offered legal services to deal with the
immigration issues that complicate HIV/AIDS for immigrants. Support groups addressed the psychosocial needs of people with HIV/
AIDS (helping people to figure out how to tell friends and family
about their HIV-positive status, role playing on safer sex issues) and
those of their family members. Former clients living with HIV/AIDS
in the "Peer to Peer" program did case management, "training people
to utilize the system." Such empowerment initiatives provide specific
examples of how activists promote oppositional consciousness.[3]

Institutional and cultural domination has impacts on interpersonal and personal levels that are also potential sites of resistance
(Collins 1990). As presented in writings by lesbians and gay men of
color, internalized oppression may exact a severe psychological toll,

commonly resulting in self-hatred and isolation (see essays in Smith 1983; Hemphill 1991; Beam 1986; Anzaldúa and Moraga 1983; Trujillo 1991). Although challenging internalized oppression has been a key element in other movements, including the Garveyite movement and the black power movement (Bennett 1984; Allen 1992), feminist movement (Echols 1989), and LGBT movement (Adam 1987; D'Emilio 1983; Duberman 1994; Deitcher 1995), there has been minimal attention to this dynamic in social movement literature. Many activists reported that an extremely important part of their work centered on creating ways to challenge internalized oppression and bolster self-images among people of color, gay men and lesbians, and women.

Outreach workers from the Asian Pacific AIDS Intervention Team (AIT) in Los Angeles created a program in response to the subservient roles they saw some Asian men playing in sexual relationships with white men, as described in Chapter 2. AIT developed an innovative project to confront this dynamic and the broader lack of positive sexual imagery of Asians in mainstream white culture. Rob, former program coordinator for AIT, explained:

> I came up with the idea, this program, "Love Your Asian Body," because I know that self-esteem is running low in the gay and lesbian Asian community. You open up all the papers and magazines and see the ads of what is considered beautiful, what is considered hot, and it's the new clone of the 1990s, the West Hollywood gay white male, and so that becomes your standard to work with. That's your standard of excellence.

According to Rob, the campaign's cards and newspaper ads provided an Asian "standard of excellence" depicting two Asians (two men, two women, and a woman and a man) in a "hot, steamy situation to emphasize loving your body." The glossy cards gave educational information on safer sex and HIV testing and advertised for events where lesbians and gay men of Asian and Pacific Islander descent could access information on HIV and AIDS.

Rob and Noel reported that there were some negative responses to the campaign from a few white gay men with Asian partners and Asian men with white partners who complained that the Asian-on-Asian focus "discriminated" against white men.[4] The idea that not having a white man "in the picture" is equivalent to "discrimination" supports Rob and Noel's framing of such complaints. Rob and Noel conceptualized these negative responses as part of an assimilationist consciousness—which relegates Asians to a subordinate social status in relationships with whites—reacting to a pro-Asian racial consciousness. Rob and Noel also reported many positive responses from Asians and Pacific Islanders, as well as some non-Asians, who felt that the images were "empowering." They also reported a significant increase in the number of people of Asian and Pacific Islander descent getting tested after the inception of the campaign.

The Love Your Asian Body campaign and others like it illustrate how social movement organizations work on the individual level to transform identities and empower people to take control of their lives. The positive, erotic images of same-sex Asian couples promote not only positive Asian American–Pacific Islander racial consciousness but also gay and lesbian consciousness. Thus, the Love Your Asian Body project provides a tangible example of building multidimensional oppositional consciousness.

One of the most powerful, widespread tactics of AIDS activism that links individual and collective action is being "out"—openly gay, lesbian, bisexual, or transgendered. Historically, coming out has been an extremely important aspect of gay and lesbian oppositional culture (D'Emilio 1983; Freedman and D'Emilio 1988; Adam 1987). Given the widespread lack of civil rights protection granted LGBTs and the prevalence of homophobic prejudice, discrimination, and violence, coming out continues to be an act of political and cultural defiance in our society (Deitcher 1995). Several people interviewed stated that being openly gay or lesbian is crucial for facilitating dialogues on AIDS and creating a safe, positive environment for those living with HIV. For many activists, this meant being "out" all the time—at social events, agency meetings, and political rallies and with family and friends.

On a collective level, lesbians, bisexuals, and gay men of color interviewed worked to promote visibility in communities of color by taking part in community events such as street festivals, parades, and health fairs. In doing so, they challenged the social construction of homosexuality as a white phenomenon and asserted that they were a part of their respective communities of color. In several cases, such high-visibility actions by AIDS activists broke through walls of silence and denial in communities of color and led to more attention to AIDS by community leaders and organizations.

For example, after being assigned a space near the end of the 1990 Puerto Rican Day parade (a common occurrence for African American and Latino/a lesbians and gays attempting to march in community parades in the 1980s and 1990s), the Latino Caucus of

ACT UP/New York broke in closer to the front of the parade. Because they entered the march early, they made it into newspapers and television broadcasts. The group did a "die-in" in front of St. Patrick's Cathedral in New York City that, according to Javier, a Puerto Rican gay man in ACT UP/New York's Latino Caucus, was a "shocking thing to do, especially in the Puerto Rican Day parade, especially in front of St. Patrick's Cathedral." They had a coffin with a Puerto Rican flag on it to dramatize the disproportionate impact of HIV/AIDS on Puerto Ricans. They also held up blown-up pictures of prominent Puerto Rican politicians with the word AIDS printed on top of them to draw attention to their lack of leadership in fighting the AIDS crisis. Even though their actions shocked many and elicited homophobic epithets from some, their signs, props, and die-ins received national press coverage, including a half-page picture in *Lucero,* the largest Puerto Rican newspaper in the United States and Puerto Rico. According to Javier, "All of a sudden we had blown AIDS out of the closet in the Latino community. . . . It was intense . . . really empowering. . . . It was the big step forward that we needed to start the discourse about AIDS in the Latino community."

Tangled up with homophobia is AIDSphobia—prejudice and discrimination against people living with HIV/AIDS. Several AIDS activists interviewed chose to be very open about their HIV-positive status. Tyrone, an HIV-positive, African American, gay man, spoke of the "triple whammy," stating that a lot of work is necessary for him and others to come to terms with being black, gay, and HIV-positive. He talked about the responsibility he and other "soldiers," who were openly black, gay, and positive, had toward those who are not out:

> Those of us who are able to be out about all of those things and have a certain comfortability around it . . . we've got to protect and nurture them [those who are not] and let them know that there is a place that they can be safe on all, any of those levels, wherever they're at, at that time and making sure they're taken care of in the process.

Clearly, this attention to nurturing and caring reflects an emotional component of activism, a component at the heart of constructing an oppositional consciousness that encompasses compassion and collectivity. Considering the stigmatization and discrimination expressed toward those with HIV and especially those with full-blown AIDS, being out as HIV-positive or as a PWA was inherently political. This is still the case today. In the year 2003, many people living with HIV/AIDS remain closeted about their status to coworkers, friends, and families.

Creating a safe environment for LGBTs, women, people of color, and people with HIV/AIDS has been an essential component of AIDS activism, according to most of the respondents, especially people of color and women. These safe spaces promoted collective identities, fostered oppositional consciousness, and encouraged people to become involved in the evolving networks and organizations of the AIDS movement. In general, empowerment initiatives support contentions by social psychological movement scholars such as William Gamson (1992) that cultural change is not merely an antecedent to collective action but constitutes action in and of itself. However, as we have seen, an individual's social position is extremely important with respect to social movement participation. Thus, cultural activism should not be initiated blindly but with careful attention to the social location of the targeted individuals or populations.

Community Embeddedness

Participating in community events as openly lesbian and gay people of color represents an attempt to forge a dual collective identity. The data indicate that such attempts to promote understanding of multiple oppressions were linked to efforts to become immersed and acknowledged in one's community. This finding is consistent with social movement literature that contends that social movement communities are linked through institutional bases and interpersonal networks (Taylor and Whittier 1992; Melucci 1989; McAdam 1988).

Interview respondents reported varying degrees of affiliation with the white gay community. People of color in ACT UP tended to have more contact with the white gay community, whereas people of color in small community-based service groups tended to have more contact with communities of color.[5] Even respondents with strong criticisms of the white gay community, who tended to work in autonomous organizations based in racial communities, noted that their organizations had links to the larger, primarily white, gay and lesbian community. Primary links took the form of subcontracting, receiving technical assistance, and using meeting space provided by primarily white organizations. ACT UP chapters in Los Angeles, New York, and Chicago provided assistance to various community-based organizations. In New York, for example, ACT UP provided the American

Indian House with start-up funding for its HIV/AIDS program. In many cases, these relationships were based upon the need for financial and technical resources that are typically in greater abundance in predominantly white AIDS organizations.

Overall, a majority of the lesbians, bisexuals, and gay men of color interviewed expressed a desire to focus their energy on work within communities of color rather than in LGBT communities per se, a dynamic that will be discussed later in this chapter. This commitment was accompanied by concrete strategies to embed themselves socially and politically in black, Latino/a, Asian Pacific Islander, and Native American communities.

One reason for connecting with organizations in communities of color was the opportunity to reach out to more lesbians and gay men. As is the case in white communities, homophobia in communities of color often causes lesbians and gay men to hide their sexuality. Although it was hoped that the increased visibility of "out" lesbians and gay men would provide a catalyst for others to be out as well, AIDS organizers realized that additional strategies were needed. Tyrone emphasized that it is crucial to be simultaneously involved in "general [black] community stuff" because not all black gays go to gay bars or belong to explicitly gay groups but are often involved in the larger African American community. Sometimes the best way to reach folks has been "under the larger umbrella." According to Tyrone, the semantics of publicizing an event are important. For example, he stated, "It's safer to come out to a 'black AIDS' event than a 'black gay' event." Tyrone asserted that being a part of the larger black community is a factor in the success of a black gay and lesbian or HIV/AIDS group. In particular, community embeddedness allows organizations to reach those who are commonly most in need of support and education. Such strategies reflected attention to the social location of potential movement participants as well as a recognition of coexisting hegemonic and oppositional dynamics in the black community. Although heterosexist culture and institutions may force some black lesbians and gays to remain in the closet, organizations and institutions in the black community provide channels for AIDS and LGBT activists to reach out to them.

Noel remarked that he has access to the Filipino community in Los Angeles because he is Filipino, speaks Tagalog, and "grew up in the 'hood." He knows the gang members, the drag queens, and their families and is considered "one of the homeboys." Marco, a gay Latino activist, stated that it was relatively easy to establish the organization

Teatro Viva, a gay and lesbian Latino/a artist organization in Los Angeles, because

> I eat at the same restaurants that my people eat at. Because I go to Burrito King. Because I go to those bars. Not necessarily because I like to sometimes, but I have to be in my community. And those are the people that should be working at these agencies. I don't think it's a secret that we're as successful as we are. We're as successful as we are because we represent our people. That's it.

Most of the activists interviewed emphasized the importance of community immersion and alliances. Strong community ties were extremely important for specific actions that may be at odds with values held by some segments of particular communities. In the face of antiaddict sentiment and community concerns with drug addiction, the People of Color Caucus in ACT UP/Los Angeles planned a clean needle exchange for several sites in the city. Frank, a white gay AIDS activist in Los Angeles, described how community connections were crucial factors in setting up the needle exchange:

> People from ACT UP/LA decided that there needed to be a needle exchange in Los Angeles and so they went ahead and did it. And they did it in a park in the black community and one in the Latino community. In the Latino community, they had enough connections and talked about this widely enough with people that they could go in and get some community organizations to actually support and kind of cover them to be able to do this. They didn't establish the same kind of relationship with the black community. And so the black community said, "You may not come in here."

Family involvement in activism was crucial as well. Teatro Viva was successful in gaining the support and active participation of the mothers of gay men. As a way to dramatize civil disobedience, mothers were arrested with their sons during an AIDS demonstration. Drag queens and their mothers organized rummage sales to raise money for a PWA coalition. The involvement of the mothers of gay men was valuable in challenging homophobia and mobilizing support in the Latino/a community.

Interview respondents also tapped into the ever-growing black, Latino/a, and Asian American gay and lesbian communities. Gay and lesbian AIDS organizations of color grew out of preexisting organizations and networks. For example, the AIDS Prevention Team in Los Angeles was established as a project of the National Black Lesbian and Gay Leadership Forum. Different non-AIDS organizations provided resources and support for AIDS groups. For example, black and Latino/a gay bars have often provided space for various organizational functions related to AIDS. In the fall of 1993, VIDA/SIDA held a fund-raiser at the Baton Lounge, a gay bar in Chicago, in which black, Latino, and white drag queens performed for free to a packed house. Activists mobilized primarily through informal social networks in gay communities of color. Many interview respondents noted that getting people out to different events was often accomplished through word-of-mouth.

Once again, the factor of intersectionality shapes the path of consciousness raising for gay and lesbian AIDS activists of color. Their "outsider within" status (Collins 1990) in communities of color leads them to challenge collective beliefs—in this case homophobic beliefs—but to simultaneously attempt to cement their ties to their respective racial communities. While simultaneously challenging and trying to fit in may seem at odds, it is necessary because communities of color are sometimes contradictory spaces for lesbians and gay men of color. On the one hand, homophobia often leads to ostracism, discrimination, and violence. On the other hand, families and communities of color provide solidarity in a racist society (Julien and Mercer 1991). Roberta, a black lesbian in BAM!, stated that lesbians and gay men of color "need their communities differently than white people need their communities because all of society is structured to make white people comfortable, and people of color generally need their communities more—for safety, for media access, for financial resources . . . and affirmation. So that homophobia matters in a different way." All the people of color interviewed emphasized their racial identities as primary aspects of their activism and their loyalty to the larger black, Latino/a, Asian American–Pacific Islander, and/or Native American communities. This social identification is translated into conscious attempts to fight AIDS among all people of color, not just gay men and lesbians.[6]

Community immersion has played a central role in AIDS activism. Activists have attempted to ground constructive dialogue and empowerment initiatives on organizational bonds with overlapping communities of color and LGBT communities. Frequently on the margins of both racial and sexual communities, LGBT activists of color have also relied on their own traditions, institutional infrastructures, and social networks to mobilize people for collective action. Community immersion strategies are critical in transforming sectors of the broader community to create more potent, inclusive challenges to the overarching power structure.

Use of Cultural Traditions

The experiences of AIDS activists I interviewed provide evidence for the theoretical argument that movement organizations make use of existing collective identities, beliefs, and cultural elements to promote oppositional consciousness and draw individuals into collective action (Friedman and McAdam 1992; Tarrow 1992). More specifically, AIDS activists root their organizing methods in the experiences and identities of potential participants—a key factor in the success of "frame alignment" (aligning potential participants' ideas of a particular social problem and related beliefs with those of the social movement organization).[7]

An important aspect of AIDS activism has been presenting prevention information and other messages in the primary language of target populations. Language barriers have frequently proven to be very serious problems within the context of the AIDS crisis. Information on safer sex, testing, treatment, and social services is meaningless if presented in a foreign language. In Chicago, New York, Los Angeles, and other cities, a primary task of AIDS workers has been translating various materials into Spanish, Tagalog, Mandarin, and other languages spoken by immigrants to the United States. It was particularly necessary for Spanish-speaking prisoners, who frequently relied on other prisoners or outside activists for translation of prevention materials, test results, and treatment information. This picture is complicated by illiteracy and more subtle sociolinguistic differences. For people with limited reading skills, activists created comic books with more simple language and pictures. In other cases, outreach workers relied on oral presentations, video, theater, and art. A gay Latino activist noted that gay Latino men in the Los Angeles area tend to be more geographically dispersed than white gay men. Many live at home, and many are married to women. They do not want to get "caught" with written information on HIV/AIDS; thus, transmitting information orally is often crucial. Jeff stressed that it is essential to provide "cultural competency training" for AIDS workers in order to make existing services more Asian-specific:

> Learning how to say "ni hau ma," which is "how are you" in Mandarin, isn't cultural sensitivity. Acknowledging that you can work with someone who doesn't know the language if you know how to use an interpreter and if you have good people skills—that's culturally sensitive, not necessarily in a patronizing "Oh let me eat your food and learn a little bit of your language."

Leonard, a two-spirited (a term used by LGBT Native Americans to more fully capture their cultural-sexual identities) Native American man, noted that many Native Americans are more receptive to "AIDS as a story." He described a few initiatives developed to teach people about AIDS, beginning with "The Grandmother's Story," an effort by five older Native American women:

> They [the Native American women] put together a story of AIDS as a creature and talked to our young people about it, and that worked, and that was appropriate culturally. And we had two gay men who put together a dance piece that was very culturally appropriate because the stories were all about Indian people and things that they had experienced and wrapping in the whole issue of AIDS.

Most organizations in the study attempted to connect with the cultural heritage of the target population as a way to promote individual and collective action. Inroads were made into black churches in Los Angeles with the AIDS Prevention Team's (APT's) fan project "Handheld." Fans, which have been distributed for many years in black churches by funeral homes and other businesses, were distributed free of charge to churches. On one side of the fan are four images of African masks and a proverb reading: "He who learns, teaches." On the other side is a list of seven different community organizations that provide testing and services to people with HIV. The fan was a culturally familiar device that served to cool off members of the congregation while simultaneously opening up dialogues about HIV/AIDS issues. The fan project was seen as a first step toward more productive relationships with African American churches.

Capitalizing on the enormous success of black film maker Spike Lee's movie *Do the Right Thing,* an APT poster declared: "Do the Right Thing—We Can't Afford to Do Less!" APT newsletters emphasized both individual and community empowerment, making use of African images and proverbs and highlighting the positive contributions of African American lesbians and gay men, such as Audre Lorde and James Baldwin, both of whom consistently expressed multidimensional oppositional consciousness through their writing and political work (see Lorde 1984; Baldwin 1961, 1972). The APT newsletter included a question-and-answer column called "The Griot"—a reference to the highly revered storytellers of West Africa.

The Asian Pacific AIDS Intervention Team handed out fortune cookies with safer sex messages in them. AIT also put condoms and lubricant in the red lucky envelopes that are traditionally given out during Chinese New Year's celebrations. The fortune cookies and red envelopes were used as icebreakers when they talked to people about HIV and AIDS. These and other tactics were used to fuse together cultural traditions and AIDS consciousness.

Teatro Viva organized a candlelight vigil and rally on Día de los Muertos (Day of the Dead). Día de los Muertos is an important holiday in several Latin American countries, particularly Mexico, and thus held special significance for many Latinos/as affected by the AIDS crisis in the early 1990s. The event served as a symbolic protest against the silence and inaction surrounding AIDS in Los Angeles. Marco linked the success of the event to the use of symbols and collective beliefs in the Latino/a community:

> The candle idea was a brilliant gesture. . . . That candle meant a lot in terms of Mexico and Salvadoran people's peace protest. It started to take on different meanings, and people were joining those marches that just believed in justice and freedom. . . . It turned into this storytelling thing where mothers were getting up and talking about their sons dying of AIDS. It turned into this really magical, spiritual, very passionate sort of thing. . . . These old ladies would get up and talk about their sons who had died and the secrets the family had about their death. And so it really started to transform how the community started to look at AIDS, but it was rituals, they were just our rituals. . . . Putting AIDS in that context broke down all these barriers that we hadn't been able to break down before.

This action represents not only activists' attention to cultural resonance and the role of rituals (Scott 1985) but collective action itself as a vehicle for increased oppositional consciousness (Klandermans 1992; Fantasia 1989). In this case, AIDS consciousness was expressed within a specific cultural context—the Latino/a community of Los Angeles.

APT, Teatro Viva, and AIT all promoted positive images of being black/Latino/Asian *and* LGBT. They held events at gay and lesbian bars in their communities. Drag shows—an important cultural tradition in gay male communities—were used to raise both funds and awareness. APT sponsored a weekly aerobics class called "Sweat at the Catch." (The Catch was a popular gay dance club in Los Angeles.) In addition to featuring APT's trademark images of traditional African masks, the flier appealed to the gay male community's attraction to the theme of sex, urging people to "Work It Till It's Hot and Wet!" The weekly aerobics class included information sharing as well as speakers on alternative AIDS treatments, clinical trials, safer sex, insurance planning, and other related issues. In the same vein, APT had "Hot, Horny, and Healthy Workshops" on safer sex. APT also developed educational materials for black lesbians, including a glossy photograph of a topless, seductively posed African American woman. The back of the card contained information on safer sex for women who have sex with women. Noel stated that outreach materials should be "simple, fun, sexy, attractive, and culturally relevant. Use gay themes." He added that it is good to be controversial: "Let's create controversy because controversy sells. I always figure if it works for Madonna, it can work for us colored folks."

In addition to creating "controversy," such sex-positive tactics have been used to challenge the antisex, particularly "antihomosex," collective beliefs that have been part of the antigay and anti-PWA backlash of the AIDS crisis. Portraying homosexuality as positive is a central part of lesbian and gay oppositional consciousness that defies heterosexist gender and sexuality conventions. This strategy is seen vividly in the "queer consciousness" that emerged in the late 1980s and early 1990s in ACT UP, Queer Nation, and other groups.

The "Divas from Viva," three gay Latino members of Teatro Viva, utilized a form of *teatro* (theater) comprising short, humorous political skits that has a history in Latino/a communities in southern California. According to Marco, the skits (performed in drag) start off "very Chicano" with "Las Comadres"—women who are gossiping about people in the neighborhood. When the audience is won over, the Comadres head into more sensitive issues around HIV/ AIDS, such as homosexuality and condom use. This includes a *ranchera* (a traditional type of Mexican song) on HIV. The Divas' *teatro* represents cultural work that simultaneously taps into LGBT and Latino/a consciousness to raise people's consciousness about AIDS and sexuality and promote individual and collective action.

Like the use of rituals discussed in James Scott's 1985 book, *Weapons of the Weak,* these cultural tactics undermine the power of elites. However, there are important differences. Although the peasant cultures of resistance studied by Scott "require little or no coordination or planning" and "avoid any direct symbolic confrontation with authority or with elite norms" (Scott 1985: 29), AIDS activists' tactics are used openly and are part of conscious political strategies that explicitly challenge homophobic beliefs and promote racial pride among people of color. Scott notes that the character of oppression shapes the form of resistance. Authoritarian rule tends to lead to masked defiance. In contemporary U.S. society, oppression within the context of the AIDS crisis encompasses racism, sexism, homophobia, and classism and occurs on multiple levels, creating the need for community-level collective action that targets multiple forms of hegemonic consciousness and inequality. Furthermore, the immediate targets are often other members of the community rather than elites. Thus, activists often rely on less confrontational tactics—constructive dialogue and empowerment initiatives—that combine community immersion and the use of oppositional culture to transform consciousness and promote collective action within communities of color.

Lesbian, gay, and bisexual AIDS activists of color devised strategies that drew on existing cultural symbols and traditions to mobilize people to take collective action. They also relied heavily on submerged social networks (Melucci 1989), such as gay Latino/a bar patrons, to create and sustain alternative institutions. What is unique about these activist techniques within the context of social movement scholarship is that they draw on *multiple* sets of oppositional collective beliefs, cultures, and networks to simultaneously challenge multiple forms of dominant beliefs, cultures, and inequalities (Tarrow 1992; Snow et al. 1986; Snow and Benford 1988). The interviews revealed multidimensional oppositional consciousness that flows out of the experiences of those living at the intersections.

Activism and Oppositional Consciousness: The Centrality of Race

Race and racism have been central forces in the historical development of the United States. In turn, antiracist struggles have had a critical impact on other political struggles. For example, the Civil Rights movement, which grew out of a tradition of protest in black communities (Morris 1984), provided ideological and strategic models for other movements, including the free speech movement, the antiwar movement, the feminist movement, and the gay and lesbian rights movement (McAdam 1988; Echols 1989; D'Emilio 1983). In turn, many of the conflicts within and between various movements in the 1960s and 1970s revolved around race. Within the data, there is evidence suggesting that the historical tradition of antiracist protest was a fundamental building block for the AIDS movement and that race has been a key factor in organizational development and strategy.

As discussed in the first two chapters, racism in dominant society as well as within many AIDS organizations affected the AIDS movement. Fierce debates have occurred regarding the most effective way of organizing to fight AIDS in communities of color. These debates occurred in both grassroots organizations in communities of color and in primarily white organizations. For example, in many cities, caucuses for people of color that had been created within ACT UP to combat AIDS within communities of color faced problems in gaining full support from the larger organization. Most of these caucuses had ceased to exist as separate entities in many chapters, including Los Angeles, New York, and Chicago, by the time of my first interviews in 1993.

Several interview respondents reported feeling frustrated with these caucuses. The experience of one African American gay man illustrates some of the issues involved in this type of formation. Mike stated that he worked hard to get people of color, primarily African American and Latino gay men, involved in ACT UP/Los Angeles's People of Color Caucus. The caucus did door-to-door educational campaigns in the black community and participated in conferences and various ACT UP actions. But the experience was very frustrating for Mike and Steven, another black ACT UP/LA member. Mike felt extremely angry because most African American AIDS activists with whom he interacted were reluctant to join the group: "Nobody wants to get involved with ACT UP." Mike was very critical of many black activists, saying that the black community is "all talk," and felt that African American activists did not want to march or demonstrate. Like Steven, he described one community-based black AIDS group as "bourgeois" and felt that they should be doing more direct action. However, he was very critical of ACT UP/Los Angeles, which he saw as often having the "mentality of a white boy's club." He asked: "Why can't I keep these Latino and black people involved in ACT UP? And it was because ACT UP was very stubborn in its ways and it didn't make black people feel any more at home than it would have been going to a Republican meeting." According to Mike, in contrast to other committees, when the People of Color Caucus of ACT UP/LA asked for money they would have to account for "every penny spent. . . . You just get tired of explaining why you spent two dollars to buy a fucking wrist band. . . . Because we didn't really have the support of ACT UP, we never really got off the ground." Mike also spoke about the risk of police brutality as a factor in the virtual nonexistence of direct action in the African American community (discussed in Chapter 5). The People of Color Caucus eventually fell apart in large part because of lack of interest among people of color. Mike's comments reflect conflicting feelings about what kind of organization would be effective in battling AIDS in communities of color; his feelings were shaped by his commitment to the confrontational queer consciousness and direct action of ACT UP but also by experiences with racial insensitivity in ACT UP as well. He concluded:

> Maybe you don't need another ACT UP because ACT UP was specifically a group of white gay men—upper class—who wanted to stop their friends dying. Because of that, ACT UP has always not been all that inclusive of everybody who's been affected by AIDS and that's gonna haunt ACT UP for a long time.

The majority of the interview respondents of color preferred to work with organizations located geographically or culturally in communities of color (as opposed to within the primarily white LGBT communities). In some cases, this preference has resulted from negative experiences within white LGBT communities and organizations, including BAM!'s departure from ACT UP/New York. However, members of BAM! and other groups often had deep organizational roots in their respective racial communities prior to involvement in AIDS work. The racial community served as a prominent reference point both ideologically and strategically for interview respondents in BAM! and other organizations. Tyrone, a member of the AIDS Prevention Team, stated that his agency's grants say "African American gay and bisexual men," but "our philosophy is community is first." Here, "community" is the black community rather than the gay community.

This preference neither precluded working with white individuals and organizations nor signaled a prioritization of fighting racism over fighting sexism or homophobia. Indeed, the majority of the activists of color tended to echo the analyses of feminists of color that multiple oppressions are often experienced simultaneously and that the prioritization of oppressions is a problematic practice (see the introduction and other essays in Smith 1983). Lesbians, bisexuals, and gay men of color interviewed consistently called for a political consciousness and strategies that strike out at racial, class, gender, and heterosexual oppression. Phil, an African American gay man, stated: "We can't compartmentalize all these things. These things are just basically interrelated. You can't look at me and deal with me just in terms of my gayness and not deal with my being an African American."

One reason for the emphasis placed on racial communities is certainly the lack of resources available in these communities, as compared to middle-class, white, gay male communities; people have put their energy where they feel it is most needed. The decision to choose race as a primary locus for political activity may also be related to the fact that people usually grow up in communities that are race and class based—particularly in racially segregated cities like Chicago, Los Angeles, and New York. Gender and sexuality cut across communities, but in general, race and class do not. Patricia Hill Collins writes that

> racial oppression has fostered historically concrete communities among African-Americans and other racial/ethnic groups. . . . Existing community structures provide a primary line of resistance against racial and class oppression. But because gender cross-cuts these structures, it finds fewer comparable institutional bases to foster resistance. (Collins 1990: 226)

As a result, gender oppression is better able to operate on the personal and family level within black communities, whereas racial and class oppressions are more likely to be countered by cultures of resistance.[8] In turn, lesbians and gay men of color have described the dynamics of homophobia on the community and interpersonal levels (see essays in Smith 1983; Anzaldúa and Moraga 1983; Trujillo 1991; Beam 1986; Hemphill 1991).

There are undeniably lesbian and gay male cultures of resistance, but they are significantly newer than racially based cultures of resistance, and people are not typically born into and raised in them (D'Emilio 1983; Kennedy and Davis 1994; Freedman and D'Emilio 1988; Adam 1987; Duberman 1994). Thus, the cultures of resistance and oppositional consciousness that are more readily available to many lesbians and gay men of color, and within which many continue to live, are racially based. This fact is vividly illustrated by the motto of the National Coalition of Black Lesbians and Gays—"As proud of our gayness as we are of our blackness"—which implies that one is more likely to already be proud of being black. The struggle in this case is to construct a collective identity that not only includes racial pride but lesbian and gay pride. Thus, racial consciousness can be conceptualized as a building block for lesbian and gay consciousness.

Other research suggests that one form of oppositional consciousness can catalyze another form. For example, antiracist consciousness acquired by white students working with the Student Nonviolent Coordinating Committee (SNCC) was a crucial building block for later student, antiwar, and feminist activism (McAdam 1988). Antiracist consciousness and feminist consciousness provided a model for gay liberation (D'Emilio 1983). Even as patriarchal ideology alienated women in the Civil Rights movement and the New Left, antiracist and leftist ideologies provided women with ideological tools to galvanize feminist consciousness (Echols 1989). However, this research focuses on communities, movements, and consciousness as discrete entities rather than overlapping and intersecting ones. In these cases, oppositional consciousness in one form is used by *another* group to develop oppositional consciousness of another kind. What is unique about the AIDS activism in my study is the community character of consciousness bridging. Racial oppositional consciousness has been used *within* communities of color to promote oppositional LGBT consciousness among people across the spectrum of sexuality.

Immersed in communities of color, lesbians, bisexuals, and gay men active in the AIDS movement wanted not only to develop a pro–lesbian and gay collective consciousness among themselves but among heterosexual community members. Throughout my data, there are numerous examples of lesbian and gay male activists tapping into racial oppositional consciousness to challenge homophobia and AIDSphobia. As seen above, they do so through constructive dialogue, participation—as openly lesbian and gay people of color—in community events such as marches, embeddedness in community institutions, and the use of racially based cultural traditions and symbols. They have used racial consciousness to mobilize around AIDS and to break down hegemonic barriers surrounding AIDS and sexuality, with the ultimate goal of building a robust multidimensional oppositional consciousness inclusive of all marginalized communities.[9]

However, racial consciousness is not automatically present among all people of color. Several respondents bemoaned the lack of racial consciousness and unity among some people of color. Yvonne, an African American lesbian, expressed resentment of African Americans who "cannot or will not confront whites on their racism. . . . Some people of color still have a 'slave mentality.'" Noel stated that many "Asian people are so toothless in terms of affecting social issues" and that there is a need to create "microinstitutions" in the Asian community in order to build more political and social power.

Expanding Oppositional Consciousness

Gay male, bisexual, and lesbian AIDS activists of color developed a rich repertoire of tactics to defy dominant ideological conceptions of the "other," transform political consciousness, and in turn galvanize collective action. These tactics were guided by four broad strategies:

constructive dialogue, empowerment initiatives, community embeddedness, and the use of indigenous culture. In support of contemporary social psychology approaches to social movements, my research
indicates that cultural strategies are part and parcel of collective efforts to undermine domination; in this case, domination takes the
form of the AIDS epidemic and the inequalities that fuel its spread.
The data support the theoretical perspective that grievances held by
individuals in oppressed groups are not consistently framed in terms
of oppression. Rather, social movement actors attempt to reframe
perceptions of social relationships in terms of oppression (Snow et
al. 1986; Klandermans 1992; Gamson 1992). Activists employ cultural elements—language, music, and historical traditions—to catalyze critical thought and collective action.

Aldon Morris (1992) writes that people are embedded not only
within cultural contexts that provide belief systems (e.g., being part
of "queer culture") but also within structural contexts that often
shape actions and limit options (e.g., being queer in a homophobic
society). Because the target populations for AIDS organizations belong to oppressed groups like poor people of color, potential participants must be convinced that participation will meet not only cultural
needs, such as feeling positive about their heritage, but physical
needs, such as employment, housing, and health care. The AIDS activists interviewed drew upon existing cultural symbols and collective identities and tapped into oppositional political communities to
create more inclusive, radical collective action frames (Tarrow 1992).
At the same time, these activists crafted their strategies with careful
attention to the social locations of target individuals and populations
in relation to systems of oppression.

What is particularly provocative is the finding that activists developed strategies that simultaneously challenge different forms of
hegemonic consciousness and oppression (e.g., racism *and* homophobia) in marginalized communities. Activists structured their efforts around multiple identities, traditions, community institutions,
and networks, as well as their own social positions and the social positions of those they hoped to mobilize. The battle over how AIDS
has been framed within oppressed communities has been complicated
by the social location of lesbians and gay men of color. They are the
"other" in more than one group, the "outsider within" described by
Collins (1990). They are of color among white lesbians and gay men
and lesbian or gay among heterosexual people of color. Conversely,
the people they are attempting to educate and mobilize can be both
supportive and antagonistic, allies and adversaries. In this sense, the

people they organize are sometimes simultaneously oppressor and oppressed.

The problem of partial oppositional consciousness necessitates collective action within marginalized communities and subsequently reduces the likelihood of direct protest against dominant social institutions, such as the federal government, that perpetuate social inequality. LGBT activists of color must address the expressions of domination within marginalized communities that exacerbate the impact of AIDS. This necessity may partially explain the paucity of direct action AIDS activism in communities of color. Activists are often so busy organizing to challenge community-level "isms," provide basic AIDS-related social services, and promote empowerment that they have less time than groups such as ACT UP[10] to protest against dominant institutions.[11]

Challenging collective prejudices with constructive dialogue, facilitating empowerment, establishing concrete ties with affected communities, and utilizing indigenous culture were (and continue to be) central strategies for LGBT AIDS activists of color. These strategies have had three broad outcomes as reported by the activists interviewed. The first outcome is individual empowerment: more people practicing safer sex and getting tested for the HIV virus as well as people living with HIV/AIDS becoming active participants in their own health care and case management. The second outcome is collective consciousness: an increase in the visibility of people asserting their racial-LGBT pride, being openly HIV-positive and challenging oppressive ideologies. The third outcome is collective action: people taking part in grassroots AIDS service projects, peer education campaigns, and social protest.

This brand of activism provides valuable insight for contemporary social movement theorists and others studying identity, political consciousness, culture, and collective action. Located at the intersections of multiple oppressions, lesbians, bisexuals, and gay men of color active in AIDS organizing stressed the necessity of challenging multiple forms of oppression—on institutional, community, and individual levels. Although community-focused activism does not always directly confront social, political, or economic elites, it undermines elite social power and empowers marginalized communities over time. Roberta cautioned against minimizing the impact of this community-level collective action:

> The actual contours and texture of what would be "activism" would be different. I think we want to be careful because we don't just

want to say that when activism happens in communities of color, it's more moderate, or it's less militant, or it's less confrontational. Because that's not always true—what's confrontational might be different.

In this instance, the methods of struggle that flowed from multidimensional oppositional consciousness encompassed economic justice, antiracism, feminism, and queer liberation. These AIDS activists galvanized a more inclusive oppositional consciousness and forged alternative strategies for fighting AIDS that can be applied in broader battles against oppression.

4

ACTing UP for Prisoners with AIDS: AIDS Activism on Multiple Fronts

The biggest challenge of all is to get our support for the prisoners.
Because you really have to have support in order to be successful
. . . and people don't get it. Society's like "Fuck those people in
prison. They're bad." So that's our biggest challenge. If we can get
the support, then IDOC [Illinois Department of Corrections] doesn't
have a chance. But right now they know we have no support.
—Jackie, ACT UP/Chicago, Prison Issues Committee

One important type of collective action is *solidarity activism*. Solidarity work involves protesting against the oppression of a social group by activists who are not members of that particular group (e.g., antiapartheid activism by people outside South Africa during the 1980s). Ideally, it is grounded in regular dialogue between those fighting from within and those outside the group. In this chapter, I examine how ACT UP/Chicago's Prison Issues Committee, a primarily queer-identified, white, middle-class group, worked in solidarity with prisoners in Illinois who were primarily working class and poor and disproportionately African American and Latino/a. Committee members were drawn to prison AIDS activism in large part because of their immersion in numerous progressive and radical social movements.

In the next section of this chapter, I examine the social position of prisoners—particularly with respect to racial and class domination. The social conditions of incarceration, marked by isolation and dehumanization, not only fueled the spread of the HIV virus within prisons but limited prisoners' access to resources and efforts to engage in collective action. Because of the severe isolation of prisoners, outside activists played a key role in raising the issue of AIDS in prison. Prison AIDS activists reported that racism and classism within the AIDS movement fostered negative perceptions of prisoners and that, as a consequence, prison issues were marginalized in the AIDS movement itself. I expand on the dynamics examined in Chapter 2 and argue that conflict surrounding prison issues within the AIDS movement reflected broader patterns of partial oppositional consciousness in ACT UP and other AIDS organizations. Those activists who focused on prison issues within ACT UP tended to be immersed in other social movement communities (Taylor and Whittier 1992) that promoted a radical political analysis of the criminal justice system and that steered activists toward prison AIDS work. In contrast, other activists with a more narrow oppositional consciousness often resisted committing ACT UP resources to prison work.

I then examine the strategies and tactics used by the committee to fight AIDS in prison. These strategies—documentation and formulation of demands, the humanization of prisoners, and pressuring elites—were guided by activist frames that connect AIDS and different forms of oppression, in particular, inequalities embedded within the criminal justice system. This activism provides another example of how multidimensional oppositional consciousness informs a social movement organization's political analysis and strategies. In addition, I analyze ACT UP/Chicago's Prison Issues Committee's use of direct action tactics and their effectiveness as well as the impact of external factors on the committee.

In the last section of the chapter, I show how this case study helps to expand the "third-party debate"—an important issue in social movement scholarship concerning the sociological roots of collective action. Although some theorists (Oberschall 1973; McAdam 1982; Lipsky 1968) argue that third-party elites (such as northern white liberals during the Civil Rights movement) are the driving forces in social movement development, others (Morris 1984, 1993; Piven and Cloward 1977) maintain that oppositional collective action is rooted in the networks, leadership, and other resources of oppressed communities themselves. I argue that the picture is more complex. The specific sociological conditions of oppression and resistance are crucial in determining how different social groups act collectively. The institutionalization of prisoners and their lack of basic human rights fostered the need for external advocacy and activism, in this case, on the part of the Prison Issues Committee. The committee was neither an "indigenous" group nor an "elite third party" but a segment of ACT UP/Chicago engaging in *solidarity activism*. Though the committee was primarily white and middle class, its members were clearly distinct from elites such as the federal government. Indeed, they were members of oppressed communities themselves, as queers and/or women as well as one working-class Latina, and represented existing social movement communities that have acted in solidarity with other oppressed groups.

The Social Conditions of Prisoners

Prison AIDS activism is relatively unique because it focuses on an oppressed population that is institutionalized. The use of the criminal justice system as a mechanism for social control is integral in understanding the dynamics of AIDS in prison as well as the place of prison issues within the broader AIDS movement. Institutionalization within the criminal justice system constrains activism among prisoners.[1] Thus, outside groups are potentially crucial in influencing social change within prisons. However, the same social forces that marginalize prisoners within dominant society also served to marginalize them within the AIDS movement.

In my study on AIDS in prison, I wrote: "The prison system itself acts as a key part of the machinery of domination—particularly racial and class oppression" (Stockdill 1995: 69). When I completed my research for this study in 1994, there were approximately 1.5 million people incarcerated in prisons and jails across the United States. Now there are more than 2 million. The U.S. rate (one out of every 142 U.S. residents)—the highest in the world—increased every year between 1990 and 2000 (U.S. Department of Justice 2001). People of color comprise about 30 percent of the country's population, yet they comprised more than 65 percent of all prisoners in 1997 (Holman 2001). In 1997, African Americans, who account for approximately 12.5 percent of the U.S. population, made up approximately 47 percent of the prison population. Latinos/as, about 13 percent of the general population, comprised 16 percent of the prison population (Holman 2001). According to the Sentencing Project (Mauer 1990), nearly one-quarter of black men aged twenty to twenty-nine were either in prison, in jail, on probation, or on parole on any given day in 1990—a statistic that in all likelihood increased during the 1990s (see Table 4.1).[2]

Table 4.1   Percentage of Those Aged Twenty to Twenty-Nine in Jail, in Prison, or on Parole, by Race and Sex, 1990

	Male	Female
White	6.2	1.0
Black	23.0	2.7
Latino/a	10.4	1.8

Source: Marc Mauer. 1990. *Young Black Men and the Criminal Justice System: A Growing National Problem.* Washington, D.C.: Sentencing Project.

Because these rates reflect the disproportionate number of whites on probation or parole (versus imprisonment), the rates for actual imprisonment are even more striking. For example, in the 1990s, the imprisonment rates for black people were 7.4 times higher than for whites (Whitman 1991). In 2000, an astonishing 31 percent of all U.S. prisoners were African American men between the ages of twenty and twenty-nine (U.S. Department of Justice 2001). Jeffrey Reiman's (1995) research provides extensive evidence demonstrating that poor people are more likely to be arrested, to be convicted, and to receive longer sentences. As a result of this and other related factors, U.S. prisoners are overwhelmingly poor. For example, 69 percent of 1991 state inmates who had been free at least a year before arrest had prearrest annual incomes of less than $10,000 (U.S. Department of Justice 1991).

Manning Marable (1983) and others contend that the criminal justice system serves as a control mechanism within a larger system of racial oppression that perpetuates the economic and political subordination of blacks and other people of color (Dunne 1989; Davis 1971; Committee to End the Marion Lockdown 1993). Marable (1991, 1983) asserts that the "law and order" mentality that arose to repress the radical movements of the 1960s and early 1970s led to the vast expansion of the prison system. This expansion continued in the 1980s and 1990s with the war on drugs, which, according to Jerome G. Miller, president of the National Center on Institutions and Alternatives, "is racially biased on all fronts and has made young Black men its enemy and the entire African American community its victim" (Miller 1992: 1; see also, Lusane 1991).

On a psychological level, the prison system actively dehumanizes inmates through the denial of basic human rights, including beatings, physical and psychological torture, and other means (Dunne 1989; O'Melveny 1989; Jackson 1970; Reiman 1995). The following

excerpt from a letter written to sociologist Philip Zimbardo provides
a snapshot of the brutal treatment targeting many prisoners.

> I was recently released from solitary confinement after being held
> therein for 37 months. A silent system was imposed upon me and to
> even whisper to the man in the next cell resulted in being beaten by
> guards, sprayed with chemical mace, blackjacked, stomped and
> thrown into a strip-cell naked to sleep on a concrete floor without
> bedding, covering, wash basin or even a toilet. The floor served as
> toilet and bed, and even there the silent system was enforced. To let
> a moan escape your lips because of the pain and discomfort . . . re-
> sulted in another beating. (Zimbardo 1985: 235)

Media-driven perceptions of prisoners as animalistic criminals
who have forfeited basic rights translate into brutal living conditions
and a lack of decent health care (Women in the Director's Chair
1994; Stockdill 1995). Within prisons, health care is secondary to the
demand for the punishment and social control of poor and working-
class people, particularly people of color. These social conditions
dictate the quantity and quality of AIDS education and AIDS care
in U.S. prisons. Kim Christensen, a member of ACT UP/New York,
writes:

> Due to their relative isolation from public view, prisoners have
> often been subjected to procedures which violate their basic legal
> and human rights. This is especially true in the AIDS crisis, where
> mandatory testing, segregation (quarantine), and other measures
> are routine in many prisons. (Christensen 1992: 139)

One Illinois prisoner wrote to the ACT UP/Chicago Prison Issues
Committee in 1994 that

> prisoners desperately need prevention and awareness programs.
> And don't you think for one minute that it is just ignorance and
> lack of money on the part of the prison administration that such
> programs are not already implemented. Instead, the bottom line
> is—they do not care. If five hundred inmates were to die tomorrow,
> the cells would be refilled before the week was out. . . . Believe
> me, these people are not in any hurry to combat HIV and the spread
> of AIDS.

This critical assessment was supported by numerous reports from
other prisoners and prisoner advocates across the country in local
jails and in both state and federal prisons.

One contributing factor to the AIDS crisis within prisons is the failure to provide condoms and other latex barriers necessary for safer sex. At the time of the study, only two states—Vermont and Mississippi—distributed condoms to prisoners. No state systems distributed dental dams—essential to prevent HIV transmission between women (Walker 1992). Prison officials have typically claimed that there is no need to provide condoms because sexual activity between prisoners is prohibited. In the words of Howard Peters, former director of the Illinois Department of Corrections (IDOC), who actively opposed safer sex for prisoners, "Sexual activity between incarcerated individuals is illegal" (Peters 1993: 1). This prohibition is clearly a product of the general dehumanization of prisoners and, more specifically, homophobia. Prison AIDS activists have pointed out that the refusal to provide the means to have safer sex has been a primary reason for the explosion of HIV and AIDS in prisons across the country (ACT UP/Chicago 1994; Slade and Sweney 1992; Stockdill 1995).

A 1990 CDC study reported that the HIV infection rate in prison (5.8 percent) was higher than rates in other public institutions, including sexually transmitted disease clinics (2.9 percent) and substance abuse programs (5.3 percent) (*New York Times,* June 6, 1992). Yet prison AIDS programs in most jurisdictions were nonexistent or extremely inadequate at best. Several of the AIDS programs developed by prisoners were actually eliminated by prison authorities. After attending the first AIDS in Prison Roundtable, advocate Judy Greenspan (PWA RAG 1993: 1) stated: "A common theme running through all the prisons was a lack of support services and education programs for prisoners about HIV/AIDS." Across the country, prisoners have consistently lamented the lack of AIDS information and services available to them (Stockdill 1995; ACT UP/Chicago 1994).

Interview respondents and other critics linked inadequate, often inhumane, prison AIDS practices to the broader role of prisons in perpetuating racial and class oppression (Women in the Director's Chair 1994; Christensen 1992). Homophobia and sexism also operate to inhibit the creation of prevention programs and provision of quality medical care. As discussed above, homophobic prohibitions against sexual contact between prisoners serve as a justification to deny condoms to prisoners. Most prisons do not have full-time gynecologists on staff—a situation that is threatening for women living with HIV. This situation is particularly disturbing given the fact that the female prisoner population more than doubled between 1990 and 2000 (U.S. Department of Justice 2001), a decade during which the percentage of total AIDS cases among women grew every year. At the time of the study, prisoners living with HIV/AIDS faced atrocious living conditions. In an article entitled "California Inmates Win Better AIDS Care" (*New York Times,* January 25, 1993), Jan Gross quotes Dan Lagano, a social worker with the San Francisco AIDS Foundation, who stated that prison staff at Vacaville (a California state prison), where many HIV-positive prisoners are transvestites, "look at them as freaks, not people." In the same article, Michael Wiseman, attorney with the Prisoners Rights Project of the Legal Aid Society of New York, declared, "Before HIV, prisons never gave good care. But with HIV, it's turned a lot of them into death camps." According to prison activist Linda Evans, the situation for prisoners with HIV/AIDS did not improve substantially during the 1990s.[3]

The severity of the AIDS crisis within the prison system led to demands by prisoners for better treatment. However, the same social conditions that promoted the spread of HIV also inhibited prisoner-led collective action. As noted by Erving Goffman (1961), "total institutions" use coercion to mold the lives of groups of people such as prisoners, mentally ill people, and soldiers. All behavior is controlled by authorities, and nonconformity is punished—frequently with violence in prisons. The relative isolation and harsh treatment of prisoners increases the costs of social protest, increasing the need for external support. Jan Speller, a member of ACT UP/Los Angeles, stated, "The population is completely hidden from view from the public. Unless someone raises the issue from the outside, the prison people treat their prisoners any way they want and no one outside will know" (Slade and Sweney 1992).

The Marginalization of Prison Issues Within the AIDS Movement

Despite the raging epidemic in U.S. prisons and jails, most outside AIDS organizations were slow to incorporate prison issues into their agendas. According to ACT UP/Chicago Prison Issues Committee members, the dominant perceptions of prisoners as second-class citizens spilled into the AIDS community. Committee members reported that racism and classism within the AIDS movement itself led to a situation in which prisoners with HIV/AIDS were either ignored or seen as not deserving of aggressive advocacy. During my work with the committee, I discovered that AIDS activists are not immune to stereotypical images of prisoners. Mainstream AIDS activists were frequently caught up in the "law and order," "three strikes, you're out" mentality that has guided our society's approach to crime and punishment in recent decades.

Consequently, the gross inadequacies within the prison system were typically not addressed by outside AIDS agencies. Many AIDS service providers across the country did not (and still do not) provide services to prisoners or former prisoners. For example, the AIDS Foundation of Chicago listed prisoners as a target population in its mission statement in the early 1990s but, in reality, did not actually have any ongoing programs for prisoners. Victor, an African American bisexual prisoner living with HIV, stated that of the five Chicago AIDS organizations he wrote in 1993 requesting information, ACT UP's Prison Issues Committee was the only one that responded. Prison Issues Committee members also stated that many organizations that provide services to prisoners and former prisoners lack the knowledge and resources to deal with the complex problems of HIV/AIDS.

This disregard for the health of prisoners is another example of partial oppositional consciousness—a powerful force that inhibited prison AIDS activism. Several chapters of ACT UP, including New York, Los Angeles, Chicago, and San Francisco, created campaigns to combat AIDS in prison. However, as seen in Chicago, partial oppositional consciousness in the organization led to a rough road for prison advocacy—both in ACT UP and in Chicago's LGBT community.

The Marginalization of Prison Issues in ACT UP

Prison issues were one area around which internal political conflicts occurred in many ACT UP chapters across the country. As described in Chapter 2, a significant number of ACT UP members, typically but not exclusively white, gay, middle-class men, were reluctant to deal with issues relating to people of color, women, and injection drug users. Carlos stated that the Treatment and Data Committee in ACT UP/New York was a very powerful group, composed primarily of middle- or upper-class white gay men with no prior political activist experience. According to Carlos, other members referred to the committee as "the right wing" of ACT UP: "It was people who only cared about developing this magic bullet to cure HIV and that's it: 'So don't talk to me about anything that is not treatment. . . . let's not deal with issues of housing, substance abuse.'" On the other side of the political divide in New York were the Latino Caucus, the Asian–Pacific Islander Caucus, the African American Caucus, the

Clean Needle Exchange Committee, and the Women's Caucus. These groups worked to expand prevention and intervention services to various underserved populations affected by HIV/AIDS, including prisoners, but often faced resistance from ACT UP/New York's relatively powerful "right wing."

Similar political divisions occurred in other ACT UP chapters. In many ACT UP chapters across the country, women's caucuses in particular have played a central role in pushing for organizational action regarding race, class, and gender, as well as sexuality (e.g., the publication of the book *Women, AIDS and Activism* by women in ACT UP/New York). In turn, women's caucuses faced resistance from many gay men in the general body. Lyle, a white gay man in ACT UP/Chicago, lamented the fact that ACT UP/Chicago had been derisively labeled as a "girl's club" by many male members, both in Chicago and elsewhere, because of its active lesbian core. During one general meeting of ACT UP/Chicago in 1994, he verbally attacked the women in the room, angrily exclaiming that they had "run the men out" of the group. One prison committee member, Kate, a white heterosexual woman, remarked: "When I went into ACT UP, I already had the perception that it was sexist because—what I had heard about ACT UP/Windy City breaking off was because of sexism, [it] was because of men that didn't want to deal with gender issues." Within ACT UP/Chicago, Carrie and Joan, two radical white lesbians and founders of the Prison Issues Committee, had a history of raising gender, race, and class issues in the organization—sometimes to the consternation of a good number of the gay men in the group.

The emergence of the Prison Issues Committee (and a short-lived committee focusing on substance abuse) between 1992 and 1995 was paralleled by the flight of several white gay men from the group. Members of the committee noted that when it began planning for a large demonstration for World AIDS Day in 1994 focusing on AIDS in prison, some other ACT UP members stopped coming to general meetings. At least one of these non–committee members connected the focus on AIDS in prison for World AIDS Day with what he perceived to be the continued attempts by women to control the group, remarking resentfully before a meeting: "Well, Carrie's got us demonstrating on AIDS in prison for World AIDS Day."

The marginalization of prison issues within the AIDS movement represents another manifestation of partial oppositional consciousness. Within ACT UP/Chicago and other groups, the focus on prison issues represented a concrete attempt to deal with the complexities of multiple inequalities. Activists with more narrow political perspectives did not see this as an effective strategy; thus, there was resistance, particularly from white gay men and activists who wanted to "work within the system" rather than "challenge and transform the system." Kate commented on the broader AIDS activist community: "In a lot of ways I don't think the AIDS activist community is any different than broader society. What I've seen is people who do AIDS activism do AIDS activism and that's it. They have absolutely no broader political agenda or concept. It's AIDS and that's it. Everything else in the world is fine."

This critical perspective was echoed in interviews with other AIDS activists in Chicago, New York, and Los Angeles and articulates the challenges facing activists seeking to advocate for the rights of prisoners affected by HIV/AIDS. Furthermore, there have been parallel patterns in other movements. For example, Angela Davis (1983) notes that within the women's movement, white feminists failed to incorporate sterilization abuse into campaigns for reproductive rights and to challenge the myth of the black rapist within the antirape movement. Davis links these movement developments to the lack of antiracist and anticlassist consciousness among many middle-class white feminists (see also Hall 1983; Giddings 1984).

The Emergence of
ACT UP/Chicago's Prison Issues Committee

Given the resistance to dealing with prison issues, how can we explain the formation of the Prison Issues Committee within a sometimes hostile organization? Like the activists mentioned in Chapter 3, members of the Prison Issues Committee (two lesbians, two bisexual women, one heterosexual woman, and two gay men) articulated political ideologies that challenge multiple forms of domination. As was briefly discussed in Chapter 2, there are two overlapping factors associated with multidimensional oppositional consciousness in the AIDS movement—prior political experience and gender.[4] Prison Issues Committee members all had prior political experience and/or were women. Kate contrasted committee members with more mainstream AIDS activists: "The entire Prison Committee is made up of people who do other political work or are aware of other political issues. There's nobody in the Prison Committee that just does AIDS work."

Kate's observation was echoed throughout the interviews and my own participant observation. Activists with no prior political experience—typically those working in large, predominantly white AIDS organizations and, more often than not, men—were far less likely to describe specific ways in which AIDS is connected to race, class, and gender. For example, in Chicago, none of the interview respondents with no prior political experience (all white middle-class gay men) mentioned the issue of AIDS in prison. These activists were also not strong advocates of ACT UP's direct action approach. Several white gay men, both in interviews and informal discussions, felt that ACT UP's disruptive tactics often did, in the words of one respondent, "more harm than good." Within ACT UP, there were white gay men who participated in direct action but were generally less likely to advocate such actions in support of prisoners, injection drug users, and other marginalized populations.

In contrast, Kate, who was active in the Progressive Student Network at the University of Illinois prior to joining ACT UP, was attracted to the latter precisely because of its direct action strategies and became a member of the Prison Issues Committee because it dealt with issues of race, class, gender, and sexuality. Her previous activism provided an ideological frame that she used to analyze AIDS in prison: "When I was made aware of the prison [AIDS] issue and looked at it, it fit into place pretty easily because I had an education behind me that gave me a basis to look at it." Janet, a bisexual white woman, had worked on different feminist issues prior to joining ACT UP/Chicago's Prison Issues Committee.

Like Kate and Janet, other members of the Prison Issues Committee made explicitly political decisions to get involved in prison AIDS activism. Ed, a white gay man who had previously been involved in Central American solidarity activism, wanted to continue doing political work on issues related to people of color and felt that, on a broader level, the issue of AIDS in prison was an important one. My own primary involvement prior to AIDS activism was in antiapartheid and antiracist political struggles, and for me, prison AIDS activism encompassed fighting not only AIDSphobia and homophobia but also the racism and classism entrenched in the criminal justice system. Political motivations merged with the personal. Both Ed and I joined the committee in part because we wanted to work with Carrie and Joan—the two activists instrumental in forming the committee. Ed stated his decision was based on "a mix of personal and political things. . . . I like them [Carrie and Joan] as people. They're a lot of fun. I also respect their thinking. . . . Joan comes out of a left background. I like that." Before and while working with ACT UP,

Joan worked on other progressive and radical political campaigns, including the Puerto Rican independence movement; the plight of political prisoners in the United States; and antiracist, feminist, and queer activism. Carrie, who identifies as a "radical dyke" and a "queer leftist," was involved in labor organizing as a student before joining ACT UP and has also been involved in numerous political struggles, ranging from working in solidarity with political prisoners to housing activism.

Six of the seven committee members had formal political experience prior to working with ACT UP. The seventh, Jackie, a former prisoner and addict, became involved in ACT UP/Chicago after finding out she was HIV-positive. Her experiences as a working-class Latina and mother living with AIDS propelled her into radical AIDS activism. Her intensive involvement in ACT UP demonstrates that radical ideology and commitment to direct action can also stem from life experiences outside the realm of formal "activism." She stated:

> When I found out I had HIV disease, I got slapped in the face with the hardest thing of all. . . . When I first found out I had HIV, it was in March of 1988; they had not even truly acknowledged women with HIV at that point. For the lack of information, for the first six months of my life, I did what the only information that was available to me told me to do: I prepared to die.

At that point, however, Jackie noted that, "I found resources. . . . Now I'm meeting women with this infection." HIV/AIDS advocates asked her to speak in public, and Jackie began to think about the potential impact of HIV/AIDS on her daughter Cristina. She recounted the pleas from women's AIDS agencies for her to speak:

> "We need somebody to acknowledge that HIV is in the women's community, in the children's community. We need somebody to talk. There's no [HIV-]positive women willing to come out." Why? Because we're afraid. What's gonna happen to our family? We're afraid of what's gonna happen to us. People are gonna ostracize our children. We're not even strong enough to defend them anymore. And I sat back, and I said, "This is horrible. . . ." I knew I had to say something. . . . When she [Cristina] gets older, if they haven't put HIV in check by then, she'll be at a higher risk of contracting HIV disease than I was shooting dope in my time.

Jackie's decision to speak publicly about her experiences as a woman living with AIDS was empowering: "I stood up, and it was like bursting out of a boulder. It was like removing 50 tons of weight off my shoulders. I stood up. I started speaking out." Within the Prison Issues Committee, Jackie provided valuable insight and leadership from the perspective of a former prisoner living with AIDS. Dialogue with prisoners and former prisoners such as Jackie was a key process that informed the committee's political analysis and strategies.

Jackie's testimony provides another example of the impact of gender in the AIDS movement and the tremendous role played by a diverse set of women. Her experiences as a woman and mother as well as a former prisoner and addict were crucial in both her understanding of the crisis and her motivations to become an AIDS activist. What is striking about the committee as well as the larger circle of activists who supported the committee by attending demonstrations and passing out leaflets was the predominance of women. Several activists stated that this dynamic is evident in other movements as well. Kate said, "In most of the work I've been involved in, the strength of the group has been in the women." Although racism and classism have certainly been significant problems within the women's movement (Davis 1983; Lorde 1984; Anzaldúa and Moraga 1983), many white feminists—particularly lesbians—have grappled rigorously with race and class and have taken steps to make antiracism a critical aspect of feminist political struggle (see Taylor 1989; Taylor and Whittier 1992; Echols 1989; Bulkin, Pratt, and Smith 1988). Ed contrasted lesbian and gay male communities: "In general, the lesbian community has taken up issues of race more than gay men."

The marginalization of prison issues within the AIDS movement illustrates how partial oppositional consciousness divides social movements. Activists developing strategies to confront single forms of domination come into conflict with activists attempting to grapple with multiple forms of oppression. In this case, AIDS in prison represents the intersection of multiple inequalities. Activists focusing on AIDS in prison bring with them models of protest from other movements—gay and lesbian movements, antiracist movements, Central American solidarity activism, progressive student activism, political prisoner solidarity work, labor organizing, and the feminist movement. The political ideologies and strategies learned in other movements were applied in the AIDS movement. For example, like Kate, my own campus antiracist activism provided me with a political critique of the criminal justice system that was useful in understanding how racism and classism contributed to the spread of AIDS in prison.

ACT UP/Chicago's
Prison Issues Committee Strategies

ACT UP/Chicago's Prison Issues Committee was formed in the fall of 1992 to pressure the Illinois Department of Corrections to improve its HIV/AIDS programs. Interviews and participant observation indicated that the committee's goals, strategies, and actions have been guided by an ideology that links HIV/AIDS to multiple forms of inequality. Below I outline three broad strategies employed by the committee: (1) documentation and formation of demands, (2) humanization of prisoners, and (3) pressuring elites. I also analyze how the theme of intersectionality plays out within each. As a group composed primarily of nonprisoners, committee members reported that their work was shaped by a commitment to work closely in solidarity with prisoners and former prisoners at all stages of collective action.

Documentation and Formation of Demands

The first strategy is the documentation of conditions in Illinois state prisons and the formation of demands presented to the IDOC. It involved conducting extensive research on HIV/AIDS-related conditions in Illinois state prisons, as well as HIV/AIDS programs in prisons in Illinois and other states. This aspect of the committee's work was a constant, time-consuming, and laborious task.

Committee members spent an enormous time over a period of three years researching the impact of the AIDS epidemic within prison systems across the country and identifying primary problems, such as the failure to distribute latex barriers (condoms, dental dams, and latex gloves); the lack of HIV/AIDS prevention, especially peer education; and inferior health care for prisoners with HIV/AIDS (and prisoners in general). This research involved acquiring information from government agencies such as the National Institute of Justice, state and federal prison systems, not-for-profit organizations such as the Correctional Association of New York's AIDS in Prison Project, newspaper articles, other ACT UP chapters, and individual prisoners and former prisoners. This research familiarized committee members with the issues and also provided models for AIDS prevention and intervention programs. ACT UP requested IDOC reports during meetings and through letters and phone calls. In several instances, IDOC refused to provide information to the organization. With the information acquired, ACT UP compiled statistics on the AIDS crisis (HIV infection rates, AIDS cases, AIDS deaths, etc.) in Illinois prisons and documented inadequacies in educational and treatment protocols (many of which existed only on paper) and practices.

Prisoner advocacy organizations and AIDS agencies were also a source of information. For example, ACT UP had a productive but short-lived alliance with the Prison Action Committee (PAC), a group composed primarily of former prisoners in Chicago. This alliance served to provide more firsthand information on health conditions in Illinois prisons. In general, other AIDS organizations in Chicago (as well as in many other U.S. cities) had little or no contact with prisoners. However, in one instance, Victor, a prisoner with HIV, wrote the AIDS Foundation of Chicago, which forwarded the letter to ACT UP. After responding to the letter, the committee established a close working relationship with Victor. The committee sent books and other literature on HIV/AIDS to Victor, who served as a peer educator, counselor, and advocate in his prison. Through weekly phone calls and letters, Victor provided a wealth of information on AIDS-related conditions to the committee. In turn, Victor directed other prisoners to the committee. This cooperation resulted in further documentation that was used to put pressure on the warden at Victor's prison, as well as the IDOC as a whole.

One of the most successful tactics in documenting conditions in other Illinois prisons was publishing an open letter in newsletters and other publications that have high prison circulations. This letter explained the committee's mission, asked for information about particular prisons, and offered to provide AIDS literature and videos to prisoners. After the letter first appeared, the committee received dozens of letters that proved to be extremely valuable in the campaign (see Appendix C for excerpts). This result attests to both the lack of information available in prisons and the desire of many prisoners to educate themselves and their friends and family about HIV/AIDS.

From this information, the committee formulated a set of formal demands and a series of educational leaflets (discussed in the next section). The demands, as presented in a 1994 leaflet entitled "(Mis)Treating Prisoners: AIDS in Illinois Prisons," were:

> 1. ACT UP/Chicago demands that IDOC repeal its prohibition against consensual sex between prisoners and implement meaningful, ongoing, prisoner-led AIDS education combined with distribution of latex condoms, dental dams, and gloves in all Illinois prisons.
> 2. ACT UP/Chicago demands that IDOC hire HIV/AIDS specialists in all of its prisons and provide all HIV-positive prisoners with comprehensive, standard-of-care medical treatment, including access to all clinical drug trials and drug treatment on demand.

3. ACT UP/Chicago demands that IDOC establish medical parole/compassionate release guidelines for prisoners with life-threatening illnesses. In tandem with such guidelines, IDOC must create extensive pre-release transition programs for HIV-positive prisoners.

Analysis of these demands and other ACT UP/Chicago Prison Issues Committee literature reveals attention to the multiple inequalities that have been wrapped up in the AIDS crisis in prisons since the 1980s. The leaflet described above also highlights the disproportionately high infection rates among people of color and women in prison (in particular, women of color). The demands for gynecologists, dental dams, and latex gloves reveal an attention to the impact of HIV/AIDS on women. The committee stressed the importance of providing treatment for injection drug use—an issue frequently overlooked by mainstream AIDS organizations and social service agencies in communities hit hard by the AIDS crisis. The committee's call for an end to the prohibition on consensual sex between prisoners (in effect, homosexual sex) exposed the link between homophobia and inadequate prevention policies discussed earlier.

While gathering information and formulating demands, committee members found that the same inequalities and social conditions that placed prisoners at risk for HIV infection also impeded prison AIDS activism. The isolation of prisoners impeded communication between prisoners and people on the outside. As is the case throughout the country, state prisons in Illinois are often located long distances from major cities such as Chicago, making it difficult for committee members to visit prisoners on a regular basis. Communication between the committee and prisoners was costly, for the only way Illinois prisoners could talk to someone outside prison is through collect phone calls. Furthermore, prisoners reported fears of repercussions for speaking out against inhumane living conditions (see Stockdill 1995). There were other ways in which the criminal justice system hindered activism. For example, when four members of the committee attempted to attend a dinner with prisoners at a nearby prison, all but one were denied entrance because one (Jackie) had spent time in prison and the other two (Carrie and Joan) had arrest records as a result of civil disobedience.

The demand that educational and support groups must be prisoner-led illustrates the committee's efforts to promote prisoner empowerment—a common theme among prison AIDS activists. The women prisoners who initiated AIDS Counseling and Education

(ACE) at the Bedford Hills Correctional Facility in New York emphasized the importance of self-empowerment ("Voices" 1992: 144):

> We said that we ourselves had to help ourselves. We believed that as peers we would be the most effective in education, counseling, and building a community of support. We stated four main goals: to save lives through preventing the spread of HIV; to create more humane conditions for those who are HIV-positive; to give support and education to women with fears, questions, and needs related to AIDS; [and] to act as a bridge to community groups to help women as they reenter the community.

The commitment of the ACT UP/Chicago Prison Issues Committee to working directly with prisoners was evident in the research and documentation phase. Letters and phone calls from prisoners provided an extremely valuable source of documentation that helped to shape the group's demands. For example, early drafts of the demands did not mention the need for support groups. After Victor stated that they were sorely needed for prisoners living with HIV/AIDS, they were added to the list of demands. In turn, when talking with prison officials and during demonstrations, the committee used excerpts from letters and phone calls to legitimize their demands (see Appendix C). Prisoners such as Victor, former prisoners such as Jackie, and members of the Prison Action Committee provided essential information on conditions in several Illinois prisons.

Communications with prisoners were also key in gathering information on existing AIDS programs outside Illinois that could serve as models for Illinois prisons. For example, an inmate in a women's prison in Florida sent a prisoner-developed AIDS education curriculum to a member of the committee, who in turn sent the curriculum to Victor, who used it to develop a proposal for a peer education program at his prison. Members of the group were in contact with activist prisoners—in particular, political prisoners such as Laura Whitehorn, Linda Evans, and Judy Clark—around the country, who shared information and gave the group essential advice.

Humanization of Prisoners

As will be discussed shortly, public officials were not receptive to ACT UP's demands, and thus the committee spent a considerable amount of time attempting to create public pressure for change. The committee targeted different communities in an attempt to raise awareness and mobilize organizations and individuals to actively challenge IDOC. A central aspect of this work was challenging dominant ideological perceptions of prisoners as subhuman.

A key aspect of humanizing prisoners was educating people about the horrific AIDS-related conditions in Illinois prisons by writing letters to the editors of various Chicago newspapers, speaking on radio and television programs, putting up posters, and so on. However, the committee discovered that merely exposing the conditions facing prisoners with AIDS was not sufficient to mobilize people. Committee member Ed stated: "The main strategy has been to publicize the issue with the hopes that people would be shocked and want to build pressure on the government to make some changes, and at this point we haven't been able to get anybody's attention." Interview respondents consistently spoke about the conservative "law and order mentality" as a tremendous obstacle to organizing around AIDS in prison. The conservative political climate of the early and mid-1990s was not conducive to organizing on behalf of prisoners. Kate asserted: "There's a very general feeling in this society that once you go to prison, that's it. Nobody gives a damn about you. You're a criminal. I know that's something I had to overcome too. 'If you're a criminal, there's really no use for you in society.' No one gives a damn what happens to you."

During ACT UP/Chicago's campaign for improved HIV/AIDS programs in state prisons, there were numerous examples of antiprisoner sentiment expressed daily in various settings. In a letter to the *Chicago Sun-Times* (January 25, 1994), Illinois state representative Cal Skinner Jr., who proposed punitive measures such as mandatory testing and segregation of HIV-infected inmates, stated: "Prisoners are not responsible people. If they were, they wouldn't be in prison. Trying to convince inmates to avoid anal intercourse and not to share needles is doomed to failure, no matter how good the 'peer education.'" An editorial in the *Chicago Sun-Times* (December 20, 1993) expressed concerns about the "confidentiality rights" argument raised by opponents of mandatory testing: "That's a strange argument to be made on behalf of convicts who have forfeited most of their civil rights by committing crimes against society." Here, a false dichotomy is made between "society" and "convicts," a dichotomy that ignores the facts that many prisoners are often unjustly convicted, most are in prison for nonviolent offenses (Davis 1971; Reiman 1995), and they *are* members of our society, over 90 percent of whom return to their communities (Stockdill 1995).

According to committee members, racism has been a key factor in the societal disregard and hostility for prisoners. Ed remarked: "It's largely a racial issue. . . . My own belief is that the whole war on crime and the war on drugs is a big backlash against primarily African Americans and people of color in general: 'If you can't kill 'em, you can lock them up.' I think it's because it's such a racially defined issue. I think it's because of that."

Thus, the committee's work encompassed not only presenting specific information about HIV/AIDS in prison but also challenging dominant ideology that relegates prisoners—implicitly blacks and Latinos/as—to second-class citizenship or worse. A crucial part of the committee's work was to attempt to "reframe" the way the general public thinks about prisoners. These efforts to reshape collective consciousness are vivid examples of the frame alignment processes presented by David Snow and his colleagues (1986). According to frame alignment theory, social movement organizations utilize specific strategies aimed at linking individual interests, values, and beliefs to the activities, goals, and ideology of the social movement organization. Frame alignment, according to Snow and colleagues (1986: 464), "is a necessary condition for movement participation."

Frame alignment strategies that center on humanizing prisoners were a salient component of the committee's efforts to gain support for fighting AIDS in prison. One incident that captures the tension between dominant and oppositional views of prisoners occurred in a discussion after I showed the video *(Mis)Treating Prisoners with AIDS* at a queer studies conference at Iowa State University in 1994. A young, female, white college student commented that prisoners are understandably not high on the public's priority list in terms of allocating resources and asked: "What if you have to choose between a mother with three children and a prisoner?" In this instance, the "prisoner" is seen as antithetical to motherhood and families in general. The dissociation of prisoners from the rest of society is again evident here. I responded, "The prisoner could very well be a mother with three children." In my response, I was attempting to continue our committee's efforts to paint prisoners as human beings with families and friends. This tactic illustrates "value amplification"—one form of frame alignment—whereby social movement organizations connect basic values (here, the importance of family) to particular events or issues (Snow et al. 1986). Jackie further explained the importance of appealing to people's sense of compassion and concern for equal opportunity:

Our world has become so callused and so self-centered. It's so hard for me to see people change. But basically I think you need to talk from the heart and you need to tell true stories like my story. I'm a success story. I was in prison. People need to be able to hear that. I mean they need to hear that on television. They need to hear that on the news. They need to get as much of that out in the open—that there are successes and that if we had a different method of dealing with people in prison we could make change.

These humanizing strategies are evident in various tactics used by the committee. The video mentioned above, produced by ACT UP/Chicago and Women in the Director's Chair (1994), centers on the faces, words, and experiences of prisoners themselves. There is no narration, and statistics and text are kept to a minimum. When I have shown the video in various undergraduate classes, it has elicited positive response from students, whose images of prisoners are typically derived from Hollywood movies and network television and who are typically unaware of the conditions facing prisoners with HIV/AIDS.

The strategy of humanizing prisoners is also seen in the various "agitprop" (agitational propaganda) posters produced by the committee. For example, one poster wheatpasted on Chicago telephone poles and bus stops in December 1993 states: "3 x-mas gifts Illinois prisoners won't get" (see Figure 4.1). Below it are three visual images representing safer sex materials, substance abuse treatment on demand, and compassionate release. Next, "Merry x-mas prisoner's. Love, Illinois Dept. of Corrections" is printed next to a coffin adorned with a red ribbon. The poster juxtaposes the humanity of prisoners—people who celebrate holidays and enjoy giving and receiving gifts—with IDOC's denial of adequate HIV prevention materials and AIDS health care to inmates.

Using the above methods, ACT UP targeted the general public through radio and television interviews as well as letters in Chicago newspapers. It also attempted to establish dialogues with state legislators. The most important frame alignment efforts, however, targeted the primarily white gay, lesbian, and bisexual community on the North Side of Chicago. The rationale here was that lesbian, gay, and bisexual communities had already developed an oppositional consciousness about AIDS. The challenge was to extend that consciousness to prisoners with AIDS. The committee found that lesbians, gay men, and bisexuals not in prison were largely resistant to connecting the plight of prisoners to their own oppression. For example, a producer at Chicago's lesbian and gay radio station refused to allow airtime for a discussion of AIDS in prison, asking an ACT UP member, "What do prisoners have to do with gays?" This false dichotomy pro-

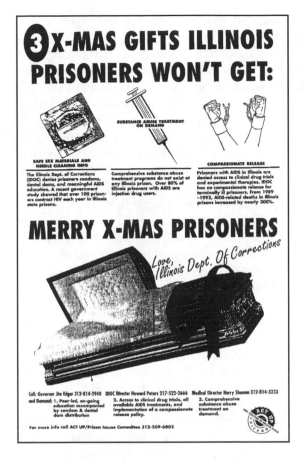

Figure 4.1
ACT UP/Chicago
LGBT Poster

vides yet another example of partial oppositional consciousness that excludes LGBT prisoners.

The committee's campaigns in the LGBT community represented examples of "frame bridging"—another frame alignment process described by Snow and colleagues (1986). In frame bridging, activists link preexisting forms of consciousness with new ones. The symbol used frequently by the committee was the red ribbon—commonly worn in the 1990s to express compassion for people with AIDS. However, the committee chose to project the ribbon as a symbol of complacency and inaction. Members of the committee argued that many people wearing the red ribbons in the early to mid-1990s did not even take the time to educate themselves about the roots of the AIDS crisis in homophobia and other inequalities and that most had never even engaged in AIDS activism. The red ribbon represented the "trendiness" of AIDS, with celebrities (most of whom failed to critique the government, the medical establishment, and the media's failure to mount a full-scale attack on the AIDS crisis) sporting red ribbons at the Oscars, the Emmys, and other star-studded events.

For the June 1994 Lesbian, Gay, Bisexual, and Transgender Pride Parade, ACT UP/Chicago members made large red ribbons reinforced with wire that they wrapped (upside down) around their necks like nooses. Their message: "Complacency and cooptation are killing us." They also carried posters emblazoned with red ribbons to call attention to the plight of prisoners and to mobilize people for World AIDS Day (December 1, 1994). Reproductions of three of the posters (Figures 4.2–4.4), which took the popular red ribbon, inverted its meaning, and challenged people to take action, are displayed below.

Similar messages and images were stenciled on sidewalks and wheatpasted on telephone poles and bus stops in gay and lesbian neighborhoods on the North Side of Chicago during 1993 and 1994. A poster designed by a political prisoner advertising the World AIDS Day protest featured a red ribbon tied around the bar of a prison cell. The text read: "Illinois D.O.C.'s program to fight AIDS in prison" (see Figure 4.5).

Another example of frame bridging was the committee's linkage between the Stonewall rebellion and AIDS in prison. In 1969, the New York City police violently raided the Stonewall Inn, a gay bar in Greenwich Village, and began to beat and arrest clients (a routine practice throughout the first seventy years of the twentieth century), who included gay men (some of them drag queens) and lesbians, many of them working class and people of color. Fed up with decades of such treatment, the queers at Stonewall fought back against the police, rescuing arrested comrades, setting police cars on fire, and resisting arrest. The rebellion lasted three days and gave

Prisoners Need

Condoms

Not

Red Ribbons!

Figure 4.2
ACT UP/Chicago
LGBT Pride Parade
Poster A

Red Ribbons

Passed Out In

Illinois:

842,716

Condoms

Passed Out In

Prison In Illinois:

0

Figure 4.3
ACT UP/Chicago
LGBT Pride Parade
Poster B

Ever Tried

Putting A Red Ribbon

On Your Cock?

Prisoners Need

Condoms.

Figure 4.4
ACT UP/Chicago
LGBT Pride Parade
Poster C

birth to the gay liberation movement (see D'Emilio 1983; Deitcher 1995; Duberman 1994). A poster used by the Prison Issues Committee for Pride Day in 1994 referred to this historical event (see Figure 4.6).

Here the committee drew upon the collective consciousness rooted in the historical struggles for gay and lesbian liberation—including the right to have sex—to raise consciousness about prisoners with HIV/AIDS. Other posters provided statistics on AIDS in Illinois prisons and demanded AIDS education, condoms, and dental dams for Illinois prisoners.

The committee was successful in gaining the support of several leftist groups in Chicago, including Queer Nation, the Coalition for

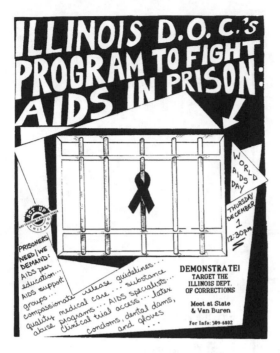

Figure 4.5
World AIDS Day
Poster

Positive Sexuality, Women in the Director's Chair, and the Auton-omous Zone. ACT UP sent speakers and showed the video *(Mis)Treat-ing Prisoners with AIDS* to these and other groups. In turn, these groups distributed the committee's literature and attended demonstra-tions. The political contacts of each of the committee members proved to be indispensable in forging alliances with other progressive groups. Frame-bridging tactics were particularly successful with these groups because their own activist work challenging homophobia and promot-ing feminist women's film and video provided them with an ideolog-ical framework within which to critique the abuse of prisoners with HIV/AIDS.

Like the activists quoted in Chapter 3, members of the Prison Is-sues Committee made use of different tactics to raise awareness and promote multidimensional oppositional consciousness. Coalitions with other progressive organizations and with prisoners were key parts of ACT UP's work as well. The participation of prisoners and former prisoners was important in consciousness-raising campaigns. As mentioned earlier, prisoner input was critical in making the video *(Mis)Treating Prisoners with AIDS,* which was used extensively to educate the public. Prisoners such as Victor provided input for edu-cational fliers and leaflets and letters to newspapers. Testimonies from

25 Years After

Stonewall:

Illinois Prisoners

Condemned to

Unsafe Sex.

Figure 4.6
ACT UP/Chicago
LGBT Pride Parade
Poster D

prisoners were read at each demonstration. A taped statement by Victor was played at the 1994 Pride Parade. Jackie, a former prisoner living with AIDS, appeared on several radio and television shows. One of the most riveting pieces of consciousness-raising materials was a pamphlet containing excerpts of letters from prisoners (see Appendix C). The following is an excerpt from a letter from a prisoner:

> I was diagnosed as being HIV-positive in 1991. I have been incarcerated since 1992. This is the most corrupt and inefficient ran prison in the state. Ex: My condition requires that I have blood work drawn every three months to monitor my T-cell count, etc. I'm also suppose to be seen by the doctor to discuss my lab results and given a routine checkup. None of the above has been done in four and a half months now. . . . When I run out of medication, it takes them two weeks to issue me more.

When Meetings, Letters, and Phone Calls Are Not Enough: Direct Action

In contrast to many of the activists and organizations mentioned in Chapter 3, a primary goal of the Prison Issues Committee was mobilizing people for direct action protest. As discussed in Chapter 1, on a national level, ACT UP became well known for its in-your-face direct action tactics that disrupted business as usual at pharmaceutical companies, government agencies, the mass media, hospitals, and other institutions. ACT UP/Chicago carried out numerous protests, including an action at Cook County Hospital in which the Women's Caucus stopped traffic by covering the street with mattresses to symbolize the beds needed for a ward for women with AIDS. (An AIDS ward for women was opened the next day.) ACT UP/Chicago member Janet commented on the direct action tactics of ACT UP:

> Instead of "Oh we didn't get this grant, so we can't do this," it's "You slammed the door in our face—we're gonna come kick it down." I like the attitude. I like the radical politic that goes with it in terms of looking at the epidemic in the context of race issues, issues around homophobia, although in practice it's not always as consistent with the philosophy as we would like it to be.

Direct action is typically preceded by a period of unsuccessful negotiations with elites. In the case of the Prison Issues Committee, ACT UP submitted a list of demands to the state of Illinois in the early fall of 1992, demanding improved state AIDS services, particularly for prisoners and injection drug users. When none of the demands were met, ACT UP organized a march and sit-in, during which approximately 200 people occupied the lobby of the governor's office in the State of Illinois Building in downtown Chicago. The December 1, 1994, sit-in yielded meetings between state agencies (Illinois Department of Public Health, Illinois Department of Alcohol and Substance Abuse, and Illinois Department of Corrections) and various AIDS organizations, including ACT UP/Chicago. Prison Issues Committee members and representatives from other organizations met with IDOC officials in the spring of 1993, but according to committee members and prisoners, no substantive changes in HIV/AIDS-related programs resulted. Subsequent letters and phone calls to IDOC had no significant results.

ACT UP/Chicago continued to gather information and establish contact with prisoners and former prisoners during the summer and fall of 1993 and implemented a public education campaign (letters to newspapers, wheatpasting posters, stenciling sidewalks, etc.). Two sit-ins at IDOC offices in January and March 1994 resulted in an interview with Carrie and Victor on WBEZ (Chicago's National Public Radio affiliate) and coverage by the *Windy City Times*—one of Chicago's lesbian and gay newspapers. During 1994, ACT UP continued to gather information—particularly from Illinois prisoners—and promote awareness in the Chicago area. As mentioned above, the focus of ACT UP's June 1994 Pride Day contingent was AIDS in prison. During this time, there were also several phone, fax, and letter zaps protesting conditions at one particular Illinois state prison.

During the fall of 1994, the committee built up momentum for a World AIDS Day protest by doing outreach to other groups, writing letters to various newspapers, wheatpasting posters, and contacting various individuals and organizations via press releases and phone calls. As in 1992, about 200 people marched through the streets of downtown Chicago to the State of Illinois Building. The demonstrators passed out information on AIDS in prison, including a pamphlet with excerpts of letters from prisoners (see Appendix C). Below are two excerpts:

> The majority of those inmates are not using any kind of protection. . . . And if something isn't done real soon the situation is going to get totally out of control. And that is why prisoners desperately need prevention and awareness programs.
>
> After having gone over World Health Organization guidelines on HIV infection and AIDS in prisons, I've noticed that not only has IDOC ignored their suggestions of condom distribution and peer educators, but also: support when prisoners are notified of test results and in the period following; effective viricidal agent, with instructions on cleaning injecting equipment; access to information on treatment options, and access to clinical trials of treatments for all HIV/AIDS-related diseases. . . . Unless the Illinois Department of Corrections seriously addresses condom distribution and a comprehensive education and prevention program, the HIV/AIDS epidemic in prisons will become far worse and more costly later on.

After marching to the State of Illinois Building, the protesters occupied IDOC's reception area, and members of the committee addressed the crowd. Angered by IDOC spokesperson Nic Howell's failure to make any commitment to substantively change IDOC practices, the group attempted to push its way toward IDOC offices to find IDOC director Howard Peters or IDOC medical director Harry Shuman. Plywood walls had been erected to prevent demonstrators from occupying IDOC offices, as they had done earlier that year. When ACT UP members and others tried to push the walls down, several rather heated pushing matches with security guards ensued, along with cursing from both guards and demonstrators. When the protesters were unable to force their way past the security guards, they stood chanting in the reception area. After a short period, a decision was made by the committee to end the demonstration, as a member of the committee declared, "We'll be back." Tactically, this decision was made because the committee had not planned for arrests on that day and because after several hours of protesting, only about twenty to thirty of the original 200 protestors remained. On a broader level, the "tactical retreat" reflected the reduction of ACT UP/Chicago's political base that had been occurring throughout 1993 and 1994.

The protest was attended by a few newspapers, radio stations, and television stations and received little coverage outside the gay and lesbian press. That reflects the power of the corporate mainstream media to filter out or simply ignore stories that expose systemic inequities (Chomsky 1988; Parenti 1988). Although Jackie did appear on *Common Ground*—a talk show on the local CBS affiliate—publicity for the demonstration was scant, and that day marked the last mass protest by the committee and by ACT UP/Chicago.

Analyzing the Committee's Direct Action Strategy

What lessons can be drawn from the protests of the Prison Issues Committee? First, it is important to examine why committee members focused their energy on direct action. Second, it is important to analyze the sociological context in which the committee's direct action took place. ACT UP/Chicago was attempting to mobilize people during a time of declining militant AIDS activism and continued political conservatism. More specifically, there was an apparent lack of oppositional consciousness regarding prison AIDS issues in LGBT communities. Committee members linked these factors to the limited impact of their direct action.

When letters, phone calls, and negotiations failed to bring about change, ACT UP/Chicago turned to direct action. Prison Issues Committee activists interviewed advocated a direct action model for two interrelated reasons. First, they emphasized that participation in direct action generates increased commitment to collective action. Second, optimally, direct action creates enough publicity to force elites to change.

Ed spoke on both of these aspects of direct action: "It's empowering to the people who are participating, and it does more than any other action to make the public think about, 'what's going on here that people take such extraordinary measures to do this?' That's what made ACT UP successful—the direct action. I think it's the best way to bring broad attention to the issue." Kate stated: "It's effective because it gets a lot more people directly involved, and if you're personally involved in an issue, it makes you more likely to pay attention to it." She contrasted lobbying that only involves a handful of people with a mass demonstration that involves hundreds. In my own seventeen years of activism, I can attest to feeling rejuvenated and empowered when participating in direct action with others. I had also learned early on that institutions do not typically redress unjust policies unless forced to do so by social protest.

The goal of direct action is to disrupt business as usual in order to force a particular agency or institution to change. Kate remarked:

> It also seems to really get to people. They pay attention. When they're in the media. When you're at the doorstep and they can't get their work done, and they have to leave their office for the day because you took over their office. And sometimes it can work just because you make yourself such a pain in the ass they just don't want to deal with it.

As Kate pointed out, media coverage is a key aspect of direct action protest. One of the committee's objectives for World AIDS Day in December 1994 was to use the media to expose the horrendous conditions facing prisoners with AIDS. However, the action was not very successful with respect to the media—virtually no television networks, large newspapers, or radio stations covered the protest. Nor was the committee successful in disrupting the functioning of IDOC offices. The campaign led to few visible changes.

From a resource mobilization perspective, one might surmise that the committee's lack of success is a result of the failure to create effective tactics. Doug McAdam (1983) argues that social movement organizations and elites engage in a process of "tactical interaction," in which elites develop countertactics to thwart social movement organization efforts. In turn, movement organizations must develop "tactical innovations" to achieve victory. The committee's unsuccessful process of submitting demands and then responding to governmental inaction with protests at the IDOC offices can be viewed as tactical interaction between ACT UP and IDOC. From this perspective, the committee may have failed to create tactics innovative enough to disrupt IDOC's daily "business" and turn public opinion against IDOC.

Kate remarked that since the 1960s, public officials and other elites have developed ways to respond to protest. For example, she noted that when ACT UP occupied Harry Shuman's office, he simply left: "When people don't respond to things, the media can't do anything with it, and they don't do anything. . . . It's been very effective on their [IDOC's] part." Kate concluded, "We need to be looking at new ways to surprise them." She stressed that activists should learn how to take advantage of advanced technology, mentioning possible strategies such as making a video to distribute to the media—"taking the news to them"—and hijacking information via computer hookups: "We have to learn how to use that." Such tactics have been increasingly used throughout the late 1990s and early 2000s, such as the use of the Internet and cell phones by the Zapatistas in Chiapas, Mexico, and by antiglobalization demonstrators in Seattle, Washington; Washington, D.C.; and other cities around the world.

Although there may have been innovative tactics that would have been more successful in embarrassing IDOC publicly or disrupting their "operations," a closer look reveals that looking at instrumental tactics alone is overly simplistic. According to committee members, what was lacking was not a particular tactical innovation but public sympathy and a broader political support base. Ed commented on the difficulty of building community support for the issue of AIDS in prison: "All along, what ACT UP has done has been to simultaneously publicize and embarrass people, and it's hard to do that here." He emphasized "the need to think through what made ACT UP successful to begin with and making some parallels between the stigmatization placed on people with AIDS and gays and lesbians and, now, with prisoners—prisoners being a group that's stigmatized, isolated politically." Direct action occurs within particular social and political contexts (McAdam 1982). Without public support, tactics—no matter how innovative—tend to have a limited effect.

Without broader oppositional consciousness around AIDS in prison, the committee had little leverage to use against political elites. When IDOC proved intransigent, the group attempted to again put pressure on Illinois governor Jim Edgar, with no success. The committee attempted to gain the support of Dawn Clark Netsch, who ran against Edgar in the 1994 Illinois governor's race. Netsch was touted by many (including mainstream lesbians and gay men) as being a refreshing, liberal alternative to Edgar, but she refused to take a stand on the issue. A lobbyist from the AIDS Foundation of Chicago defended Netsch, claiming that taking a supportive stance on prisoners with AIDS would only "hurt her campaign." The lobbyist also claimed that Netsch was "very supportive in private" and would take action if elected. Reflecting the committee's confidence in Netsch, one ACT UP member called these comments "Bullshit." Regardless of Netsch's level of commitment to prisoners, neither Edgar or Netsch felt it necessary to address the issue during their respective campaigns. ACT UP activists felt that candidates ignored the issue largely because the voters did not see the rights and well-being of prisoners as important. This attitude reflects the broader challenge for any activists attempting to organize in support of prisoners in a political climate in which prisoners have been monolithically (and inaccurately) portrayed as violent criminals.

The activists frequently came back to the lack of compassion for prisoners as a core obstacle to their work. At the beginning of this chapter, Jackie mentioned the committee's primary challenge: to get support for prisoners. She went on to say: "The second biggest challenge will be to get IDOC to change. That's not the first biggest challenge. That's the second biggest challenge. And sometimes I think we work backwards. So we're almost making ourselves take longer." Jackie's comments reflect the importance of building a strong political base of support. It requires a transformation of consciousness—in this case, reconceptualizing prisoners as human beings who deserve health care and other services. Thus, the frame alignment issues discussed in the section above are critical.

One particular issue raised by committee members was the process of deciding which segments of the public to target for consciousness raising and what strategies to use. Jackie argued that the committee needed to reach out to the communities from which most prisoners came:

> If we want to do something good in the prisons, we have to go to the poor people. We have to go to the neighborhoods that are being impacted. But not just go there and give them street theater and that, but also tell them how they can be effective. And you really have to carry them by the hand because like the PISD [ACT UP/Chicago's People with Immune System Disorders] caucus, people who are very poor may not have time to do the work themselves. They would dedicate a signature and the name, but they may not pay that stamp to mail it.

Here Jackie raises the thorny issue of "outside" activists going into other communities to organize. Other members of the committee felt that it would be inappropriate for the primarily middle-class, white committee to focus on organizing in poor and working-class communities, especially communities of color. As a former prisoner living in a working-class Latino/a community, Jackie connected on several levels with prisoners and their families. But the bulk of the committee occupied different socioeconomic and racial positions and felt that organizing in working-class and poor communities of color could potentially be elitist and paternalistic. The activists' recognition of race and class differentials was an important factor in their work. Ed commented, "And then of course that [organizing in communities of color] presents an obstacle for us as mostly a white group, and there's also the obstacle of making contacts with prisoners." Thus, mobilization strategies are shaped by activists' beliefs on how best to work, given their particular positions within systems of oppression.

In hindsight, the committee, if not beset with its own internal disintegration, might have continued to build relationships with prisoners, former prisoners, and other organizations working on prisoner rights. Such alliances might have proved sufficient to balance the racial and class privilege of the committee. In addition, there may have been other ways to raise consciousness in Chicago's LGBT communities. However, it would have been difficult, given the fact that in 1995, the committee and ACT UP/Chicago ceased to exist.

The committee's disintegration in 1995 in large part paralleled the disintegration of ACT UP/Chicago, which had begun as early as 1992 and was linked to illness and death, burnout, internal conflict (see Chapter 2), less media coverage of AIDS activism, the bureaucratization of AIDS (ACT UP members finding jobs in mainstream AIDS agencies), and repression (see Chapter 5). In addition to these factors, personal factors led to the demise of the committee. Janet had actually left the committee in 1994 to pursue activism in another group. In turn, Kate left the group and, like Janet, moved into other areas of radical political organizing. Joan and Ed both faced increased pressures at work and attended meetings less and less. In February 1995, as the remaining members tried to maintain contact with prisoners, I found out that I had been infected with HIV, which required that I take time out to take care of myself for several months. With Jackie battling AIDS and raising a young daughter, the bulk of the committee's work was left to Carrie. Although Carrie, Jackie, and I continued to provide information and emotional support to individual prisoners at several prisons in 1995 and 1996, the committee, along with ACT UP/Chicago, no longer existed.

* * *

Although the Prison Issues Committee did not force an overhaul of HIV/AIDS-related programs and policies in the Illinois Department of Corrections, there were concrete successes. ACT UP's letters; exposés; phone, letter, and fax zaps; and demonstrations forced IDOC to make changes, albeit often minimal ones. For example, pressure

from the committee led to the hiring of one IDOC AIDS peer educator. That was a hollow victory, given the fact that the former prisoner
was the only such educator for the entire state prison population that
numbered in the tens of thousands, but it was a positive change none-
theless. External pressure combined with the committee's support for
Victor and other prisoners led to the establishment of a peer education program—spearheaded by Victor—at his prison. Other smaller
but important victories also occurred. In several cases, the committee
was able to push medical staff at Victor's prison to provide more
competent care for inmates with HIV/AIDS. For example, after the
prison stopped providing prisoners with HIV/AIDS with the dietary
supplement Ensure, the committee forced the prison to reinstate its
distribution.

Another critical outcome was the committee's role in helping
prisoners to push for changes from the inside. Despite its miniscule
budget, the committee sent in hundreds of educational pamphlets, articles, books, and other materials. Prisoners consistently reported that
reading them was very empowering, whether they applied this
knowledge for their own health or the health and well-being of their
fellow inmates. Committee members also provided legal, medical,
and sexual assault referrals for prisoners and former prisoners.

As described throughout this section, prisoners, though physically unable to attend direct action events, did participate indirectly
in direct action events. Their testimonies were read, and in one instance played over a sound system (Chicago's LGBT Pride Parade,
1994), at demonstrations and rallies. The information they provided
was used to develop the demands issued to public officials when
ACT UP members occupied the IDOC reception area and offices. As
mentioned earlier, a political prisoner designed the flier advertising
the World AIDS Day demonstration. Former prisoners and committee
member Jackie spoke at many of the protests, as did other former
prisoners from the Prison Action Committee.

Expanding the Third-Party Debate

AIDS in prison activism provides insight into debates on the role of
third parties in social movement development and outcomes. One
perspective on third parties contends that social movements are
dependent on outside groups for money and resources (McAdam
1982; Oberschall 1973; Lipsky 1968). According to this viewpoint,

oppressed groups lack the organizing skills and resources necessary for effective collective action and seek assistance from outside elites, including government agencies and leaders, courts, affluent liberals, and philanthropic foundations. This perspective was common among early resource mobilization analyses.

Aldon Morris's work on the Civil Rights movement challenges this third-party thesis, demonstrating that "the majority of local movements were indigenously organized and financed" (1984: 281; see also Morris 1993). Morris presents an indigenous model in which social movements are organized by indigenous groups and are reliant on indigenous resources. Sustaining a movement depends on the community having basic resources, such as organizations, networks, leadership, money, and participants. Outside help is helpful but is not "a causal determinant" (Morris, 1984: 283). Morris distinguishes between two kinds of outside resources: "A distinction must be made, however between resources voluntarily supplied by individuals and groups who identify with the goals of the movement and those supplied by political actors (e.g., heads of state, courts, national guards) in response to political crises created by the movement" (Morris 1984: 286). The former "facilitate the social change efforts of the dominated community." The latter are not assistance but outcomes brought about by social protest. He goes on to argue that both types of responses "depend on the strength of an indigenous movement and the scope of change it seeks" (Morris 1984: 286).

My research indicates that neither of these perspectives captures the collective action of ACT UP/Chicago's Prison Issues Committee. Prison AIDS activism, in this case, was not primarily "indigenous," nor was it led by "outside elites." This collective action can be more accurately described as *solidarity activism:* social movement activities that are conducted by "outside activists" (not elites) and are guided by dialogue between the "outside activists" and "inside activists." Solidarity work is shaped by three interrelated social factors: (1) the social position of the dominated or inside group, (2) the social position of the outside activists, and (3) the relationship between the inside and outside groups.

As an institutionalized, multiply oppressed population, prisoners face great obstacles in creating effective protest campaigns. They are poor and disproportionately people of color, and they are locked up—physically isolated. These social conditions severely reduce their access to resources and impede activism. These particular conditions create the need for outside support. Former prisoner Jackie remarked,

As an ACT UP member, I feel totally like what we're doing is the most important thing because . . . AIDS is a horrible thing, AIDS in every way, shape and form—economically, socially—you mention it, AIDS is a terrible thing. But the thing that I see that's most atrocious going on right now is the fact that AIDS is so hidden in the penal system, and it's so untouchable. I think it's the thing that needs to be addressed right now.

Members of ACT UP's Prison Issues Committee identified the need for solidarity work on behalf of prisoners living with HIV/AIDS. Because they were primarily middle-class "nonprisoners," the committee was not "indigenous." However, it would be inaccurate to call the committee an "elite third party." Although most committee members had white racial and middle-class privilege, they were oppressed as queers or women or both. As a confrontational, queer organization, ACT UP challenged established political institutions and, in many cases, was also in conflict with mainstream, assimilationist segments of the LGBT community. Furthermore, as shown in Chapter 5, ACT UP faced repression from the police, the criminal justice system, and the Federal Bureau of Investigation (FBI). The committee was an outside solidarity group providing various resources and support to prisoners, not a "third party." It was the committee itself that acted in opposition to dominant social institutions, specifically the Illinois Department of Corrections.[5]

One central social characteristic of the committee was that its members were immersed in long-standing, progressive political communities. Each member of the group had been involved in radical and progressive politics for anywhere from five to twenty years. Thus, they were different from frequently mentioned third parties, such as liberal sectors of the federal government during the Civil Rights movement.

Of particular interest here is the prominent role that queer-defined lesbians have played in the AIDS movement. Carrie, one of the many self-described "radical dyke" AIDS activists, described her political consciousness as "leftist, antiracist, queer, feminist, and pro-sex."[6] Although heterosexual women played important roles in ACT UP, my interviews and participant observation indicate that radical lesbians in particular were pivotal players in the development of more inclusive, leftist strategies in ACT UP chapters in Chicago and in other cities. In particular, they helped many ACT UP chapters to expand their AIDS consciousness to challenge AIDS at the intersections—including HIV/AIDS among women, people of color, injection drug users, and prisoners. Such queer feminists spearheaded committees on substance abuse and prison issues in ACT UP/Chicago. Women, particularly lesbians, in ACT UP/Los Angeles and ACT UP/San Francisco provided leadership in the campaign to confront the horrific conditions facing prisoners with HIV/AIDS in California (Slade and Sweney 1992) and in New York (ACT UP/New York 1992). This activism was driven by ideology, strategies and tactics, and alliances developed through immersion in other social movement communities. The profound impact made by "radical dykes" on the AIDS movement illuminates the impact of queer feminism in connecting different political struggles—on both ideological and strategic levels.[7]

Skills and networks developed while working in the feminist movement, the LGBT movement, and other movements were used by the Prison Issues Committee. The radical lesbian feminist community and other social movement communities also provided access to other activists and organizations, tactical repertoires, fax machines, video-making expertise and equipment, and so on. These resources were used not only to put pressure on IDOC but to provide prisoners with support. Jackie reported:

> The most wonderful thing that our prison committee is doing right now is the support that we're giving to the prisoners via letters and mail and newsletters and making them aware that we're gonna have this demo for them. . . . That's the best thing we can do. Even if the prison committee ceased to exist, it's imperative that Victor continues having his support because that would just be one more support that just disappeared—poof—from him. And it would not be a good thing. It's the most wonderful thing we're doing right now, but do we realize how much we are responsible for these people now? We have to.

ACT UP's support for prisoners is evidenced in Victor's letter to one of Chicago's gay and lesbian newspapers. In turn, Victor extended his support, encouraging readers to participate in ACT UP's 1994 World AIDS Day demonstration:

> I've learned that I'm not just a person with HIV, but a person *living* with HIV and that there are people and organizations who've taken it upon themselves to offer their services to help us live with this virus, such as ACT UP/Chicago's Prison Issues Committee, who have gone more than the mile to stand in the gap for us—who not only have to battle against HIV/AIDS, but also the ostracism of Mr. John Q. Public. It is for these reasons we [prisoners affected by HIV/AIDS] urge you to support ACT UP on World AIDS Day.

As described earlier, most committee members expressed a concern that they remain cognizant of their own race and class privilege as well as their nonprisoner status. At the same time, Jackie injected the perspective of a former prisoner living with AIDS. The committee prioritized the input of prisoners and strived to work closely with prisoners and former prisoners at each step of the collective action process. The committee not only provided information and other resources that helped prisoners on an individual level but also assisted them in taking action themselves. Ed stated that a critical goal "is trying to empower prisoners." That was done by having active dialogues with prisoners and asking them what they needed and what kind of action the committee should be taking. Committee members expressed that they wanted to avoid paternalistic situations in which they attempted to decide what was best for prisoners in terms of HIV/AIDS.

This ideological perspective led to close alliances with prisoners and former prisoners, as described throughout this chapter. These alliances have included the partnership between the committee and the Prison Action Committee, communication with individual prisoners and former prisoners in Illinois and other states, extensive input from prisoners into the making of the video *(Mis)Treating Prisoners with AIDS*, letters written by prisoners to newspapers, and prisoner testimonies read at demonstrations.

Despite these successful collaborative efforts, the conditions of incarceration made working directly with prisoners very challenging. The committee found it difficult to establish contact with prisoners. Obviously, prisoners could not attend the protests. In other states, prisoners have staged protests inside while ACT UP has held a demonstration outside the prison. For example, HIV-infected inmates staged hunger strikes and medication strikes to protest conditions at California's state prison at Vacaville. ACT UP's support and involvement led to legislative investigation and subsequent improvements in AIDS care (Slade and Sweney 1992; ACT UP/Chicago 1994). However, ACT UP/Chicago did not develop strong enough relationships with a group of prisoners at a particular prison to be able to do that.

* * *

The Prison Issues Committee focused its energy on two interconnected strategies: transforming public consciousness around the issue of HIV-positive prisoners and putting pressure on the Illinois

Department of Corrections to improve its HIV/AIDS programs. A key element of the committee's work was challenging partial oppositional consciousness within the gay and lesbian community—especially racist and classist perceptions of prisoners. Humanizing prisoners in the eyes of the general public and, more specifically, the gay and lesbian community was at the core of the committee's work. ACT UP activists attempted to tap into basic social values as well as queer and AIDS consciousness to transform the way people think about prisoners. Activists used symbols such as the red ribbon and, as mentioned in Chapter 3, tapped into themes of sexual liberation within LGBT culture.

In contrast to Chapter 3, this chapter has focused on direct action activism. However, both chapters show how multiple forms of social inequality are woven into the AIDS crisis and how activists challenge them. Both chapters illuminate some of the connections between intersecting oppressions, collective consciousness, and collective action. In this chapter, activists attempted to challenge dominant ideological frames, thereby promoting multidimensional oppositional consciousness that was essential for mobilization around AIDS in prison. They did so by linking queer and AIDS consciousnesses to build an antiracist and anticlassist consciousness. This chapter also illustrates the impact of one social movement community (radical lesbians) on another movement (the AIDS movement). Chapter 5 examines the impact of repression on the different forms of grassroots AIDS activism, including the collective action examined in Chapters 3 and 4.

5

Cops, Courts, and the FBI: Repression and AIDS Activism

Our protests are limited to the civil rights thing. . . . We ain't goin'
out there and throwin' no blood on nobody and chain linking ourselves to no fences to be shot and killed. That's not happenin'.
　　　　　　　　　—Tyrone, AIDS Prevention Team, Los Angeles

They [the Chicago police] went right through the middle of us with
horses and they just started hitting people right in the crowd. . . .
I'm very afraid of them, and that's their strategy.
　　　　　　　　　　　　　　　　　—Jackie, ACT UP/Chicago

The words of AIDS activists Tyrone and Jackie illuminate the impact
of repression, both expected and actual, on AIDS activism. Brenda
Uekert defines repression as "the use or threat of use of coercion by
governing authorities to control or eliminate opposition" (Uekert
1994: 4). For this chapter, this definition will be expanded to include
any actions taken by government authorities (or other elites) to impede mobilization of social movement participants; harass and intimidate activists; divide organizations; and physically assault, arrest,
imprison, and kill movement members. My analysis shows how repression affects strategic decisionmaking among social movement
participants, intimidates activists, contributes to organizational demise, and hinders coalition building. The data also indicate that systems of racial, class, and heterosexual inequality facilitate repressive
responses to progressive social movements.

According to McCarthy and Zald (1973: 26), elites take two general approaches to exert social control over oppositional movements. The first approach is characterized by facilitation—negotiations, concessions, support, cooptation, and forming coalitions—which aims to control the "direction of dissent." The second approach is aimed at "minimizing dissent" (see also Oberschall 1973). In this chapter, I deal specifically with the second approach—repression as defined above—although it is important to note that authorities often respond with repression and negotiation or cooptation simultaneously (Allen 1992; Piven and Cloward 1977).[1]

Klandermans contends that "the willingness to participate in a social movement is a function of the perceived costs and benefits of participation" (Klandermans 1988: 583). These costs may include time, energy, financial contributions, job loss, stress, harassment, and arrest (Fantasia 1989; Churchill and Vander Wall 1990).[2] In turn, people are motivated by tangible "benefits" (passage of a particular piece of legislation, improved living conditions) as well as less tangible motivations (anger, hope, love, indignation, desire for justice). High levels of repression (surveillance, violence, incarceration, assassination) raise the costs of movement participation and may intimidate activists, hindering the emergence of collective action or causing activists to withdraw from power struggles (Tilly 1978).[3]

In the following sections, I examine how the combined weight of three interrelated factors had a debilitating effect on the AIDS movement between 1987 and 1994: (1) knowledge, particularly among activists of color, of historical political repression of other antiracist social movements; (2) contemporary perceptions of the criminal justice system as racist and classist, particularly among activists of color; and (3) political repression, often within the context of homophobia, targeting ACT UP. These factors discouraged direct action tactics; used up valuable time, energy, and resources; and created fear, stress, and mistrust. Furthermore, the social locations of activists in relation to systems of oppression influenced their expectations of repression, their strategic decisionmaking, and their experiences with repression.

COINTELPRO and Rodney King: Legacies of Fear

Activists of color in Los Angeles, New York, and Chicago—both in ACT UP and other groups—were much more likely than white activists to perceive political repression to be a real threat in the United States during the 1980s and 1990s. The expectation of police violence, arrests, imprisonment, and deportation is one variable that weighed into the decision to participate in collective action, particularly civil disobedience. The interview data indicate that collective memories of past government attacks on radical antiracist struggles during the 1960s and 1970s, along with expectations of racist and classist treatment by the police and the courts, discouraged confrontational AIDS protest among many, but by no means all, people of color interviewed.

Collective Memories of Repression

The interviews show that collective memories have been produced by the extreme deception and violence used by the federal government and other authorities to crush the radical movements of the 1960s and 1970s—especially those led by people of color. Comments, particularly from African Americans and Puerto Ricans, about the potential for government reprisals against AIDS activism were framed within this larger historical context.

The majority of AIDS activists of color spoke specifically about the U.S. government's efforts to destroy the black power movement and other movements for justice and equality, such as the American Indian Movement (AIM) and the Puerto Rican independence movement. This repression is well documented. Several AIDS activists interviewed specifically mentioned the FBI's Counter Intelligence Program (COINTELPRO) unit that worked to thwart the Communist Party in the 1950s and exerted its greatest efforts in the late 1960s and early 1970s to crush the Black Panther Party by fabricating evidence used to imprison activists, infiltrating organizations, forging correspondence, conducting surveillance, and killing dozens of radical activists (Churchill and Vander Wall 1990; McAdam 1982, 1988; Glick 1989; O'Reilly 1989; Shakur 1987).

Repression was a significant factor in the demise of the Black Panther Party, a group that worked to challenge police brutality and other forms of institutionalized racism as well as to promote empowerment in poor and working-class African American communities. Violence, intimidation, harassment, and surveillance increased the risks of participation in the organization, making it difficult to recruit new members. Trumped-up prosecution and false imprisonment of Panther leaders (e.g., Geronimo Pratt and Huey P. Newton) led to costly and time-consuming legal battles. Fear of informers generated suspicion and distrust that precipitated internal conflict. Leaders such as the charismatic Fred Hampton, chairman of the Black Panther Party in Chicago, were murdered in cold blood by the local police, working in collaboration with the FBI. Overall, these state responses undermined support within the black community, leading to a shift from community organizing to defending the organization from outside attacks (Allen 1992; Churchill and Vander Wall 1990; Helmrich 1973; Killian 1975; Marx 1974; McAdam 1982). Other organizations and movements were targeted with this calculated terrorism as well. The FBI has been implicated in the assassinations of key leaders of AIM in the 1970s, including Pedro Bissonette, Byron DeSersa, and Anna Mae Aquash. AIM member Leonard Peltier has been incarcerated since 1976 as a result of the FBI's intimidation of key witnesses, tampering with evidence, and outright perjury, all of which led to his conviction on murder charges (Churchill and Vander Wall 1990).

It is from this perspective that activists of color spoke about the possibility of repression for direct action AIDS activism. Stephanie, an African American lesbian in ACT UP/Chicago, spoke about the police and the FBI: "History has shown us that they're not gonna show us any mercy. And there's nothing that I or anybody else can do to lessen that fear because that is a reality." Maria, a Puerto Rican activist, said she would not risk arrest in an AIDS protest because this would amount to "giving the government some kind of information about myself," such as fingerprints and photographs that could be used against her in the future.

While discussing the role of direct action, Tyrone, an African American gay man with the AIDS Prevention Team in Los Angeles, stated that the mere presence of a large group of black people "makes people nervous" and often leads to negative reprisals. The following quote reveals how knowledge of past repression influences contemporary expectations of repression:

> If we had been the ones who formulated the ACT UP model, it wouldn't be as successful as it is today because what would happen is we would be still in jail. A lot of us would be dead. . . . We're fortunate in that we do have the ACT UPs to go out and do it. 'Cause if it wasn't for fear that we would get knocked in the head and beat up or whatever, we would be doing the same thing, but what's real historically for us is that when we act up we get shot and killed or we get institutionalized for the next twenty-five, thirty years. I don't think people are at that point with AIDS and HIV that they're willing to take that risk.

This sentiment was shared and expressed in strikingly similar language in several other interviews. The sheer brutality targeted at radical activists in the 1960s and 1970s is seared into the memories of many activists today, particularly African Americans and Latinos/as.

Contemporary Expectations of Repression

Expectations of repression were articulated not only within the context of historical repression but within the context of contemporary racism and classism in the criminal justice system. Activists' perceptions of a greater possibility of police brutality, arrests, conviction, and longer sentences for people of color are borne out by research on the criminal justice system (Abu Jamal 1995; Bridges and Crutchfield 1988; "Special Section" 1998; Gray 1991; Mauer 1990; Reiman 1995; *Stolen Lives* 1999). These patterns of injustice affected strategic choices and in particular operated as a deterrent to civil disobedience among activists of color working outside ACT UP. Whites interviewed who did *not* engage in direct action did so for different reasons than people of color. These white respondents' decisions were based primarily on a sense of propriety and a belief that working within the system is appropriate and adequate. For example, Angelo, a white gay AIDS prevention worker, expressed doubts that ACT UP/Chicago's participation in the annual Pride Parade "had the right impact. . . . Every Gay Pride [Parade], the only thing the press shows is the drag queens and the people causing problems [ACT UP]. They don't show the professors, the lawyers, the doctors that are gays and lesbians."

Several respondents of color expressed a feeling that many white activists were not aware of the greater potential for repression against people of color engaging in protest. This perspective is supported by the interviews with white activists—with the important exception of leftists in ACT UP. Phil, an African American gay male AIDS activist in Los Angeles, stated:

> I think it's important to say . . . that there sometimes has been an expectation that people of color ought to be protesting in ways that we're supposedly not doing. But I think that one needs to look at the way the criminal justice system deals with people of color and to recognize what role that plays in people's decisions as to how they're gonna participate, whether they're gonna participate.

Such comments were frequently made in reference to ACT UP's confrontational tactics (stopping traffic, sit-ins). Although all the activists of color acknowledged the importance of such tactics in numerous successes in the AIDS movement (primarily actions by ACT UP), most of the activists of color *not* in ACT UP expressed a reluctance to encourage such tactics in communities of color.

Police brutality was by far the most frequently discussed aspect of the criminal justice system by respondents. Virtually all the respondents of color expressed fear of police violence in response to direct action protest. Several respondents reported being the victims of police abuse, both during political demonstrations as well as routine interactions on the street (such as during a traffic stop). My first interviews were conducted in Los Angeles in the wake of the 1992 rebellion following the acquittal of the police officers who savagely beat Rodney King, a young African American man, in 1991. Frank, a radical white gay activist in Los Angeles, noted that immediately following the verdict, there were heated discussions among black activists as to whether they should go to Simi Valley (the affluent, primarily white Los Angeles suburb where the trial was held) to protest the verdict along with ACT UP/Los Angeles. Frank recounted that some members of black lesbian and gay organizations felt that the "danger was much too great" for blacks to engage in civil disobedience. Others spoke in favor of civil disobedience. The anxiety over police brutality was expressed in other cities and in other communities of color as well. Catalina, a Latina activist and caseworker at an AIDS agency in Detroit, linked police brutality to the fear of social protest: "Not being able to trust the police is a huge problem in the Latino community. There is a sense of betrayal. The police represent protection—but they've violated this. . . . I think people are afraid of protesting 'cause of the police."

Because of the minimal amount of direct action taken, there were virtually no instances in the data of police abuse targeting AIDS activists of color who were not participating in ACT UP demonstrations. The vast majority of the instances of police violence and harassment in this study targeted members of ACT UP (both white people and people of color). It is difficult to discern whether police targeted protestors of color more than white protestors during ACT UP demonstrations. Elena, a Puerto Rican activist with VIDA/SIDA (an alternative health clinic for people with HIV/AIDS in Chicago), was thrown headfirst by police into the side of a Chicago police paddywagon during an ACT UP/Chicago demonstration, but this treatment was typical of the level of police violence meted out to white ACT UP protestors during the late 1980s and 1990s. Steven and Jack, both African American gay men, felt they were singled out by police at predominantly white AIDS protests. Steven, a member of ACT

UP/Los Angeles, maintained that at demonstrations, "cops would jump over twenty white boys to get to me." In contrast, Stephanie noted that being arrested with white people lessened the probability of her being brutalized:

> I've been very lucky. . . . I think part of some of the reasons that I'm not treated as bad as [white protestors]. . . . They can beat the shit out of a lot of white people and not touch me, and that has been the case a number of times. . . . It would be so obvious. It's complicated. Sometimes it works to my advantage. Then there are times when they're beating everyone up.

It is certainly possible that both dynamics exist. In some situations, the police may perceive a risk in targeting and abusing the only people of color at a mostly white protest; but in other situations, the police may automatically perceive people of color as more threatening or disruptive. There is also the possibility of a gender effect. The police may be more likely to beat black men than black women. Unfortunately, the findings in my study do not allow for any definite conclusions regarding the differential treatment of people of color at ACT UP actions.

What is clear from the data is the impact of expectations of police brutality. Stephanie commented that, "It would definitely be different if I were getting arrested with a bunch of black people instead of a bunch of white people." Stephanie's comments reflect a common sentiment among activists of color—both in ACT UP and other groups. Donald stated that if the People of Color Caucus of ACT UP/Chicago had been larger and stronger, it would have been repressed by authorities. The largest people of color caucus in the study, the Latino Caucus of ACT UP/New York (thirty to forty people at its peak), experienced police and possibly FBI harassment (described in the next section). Maria asserted: "If ACT UP would have been only black men or Puerto Rican or Chicano men organizing in their community, and there was no white face or no light skin, and they would be gay, radical queer transvestites, gay men organizing, they would have been lynched like [black] people were lynched in the South in 1875." This belief is supported by the extensive documentation of past and current police violence targeting black, Latino/a, and Native American activists, as well as nonactivists murdered in cold blood by the police, such as Anthony Baez, Mario Paz, and Tyisha Miller (see Davis 1971; Marable 1983). For example, Amadou Diallo, a twenty-two-year-old immigrant from Guinea (a West African country), was in the vestibule of his apartment building in the Bronx on February 4,

1999, when four white New York City police officers fired forty-one shots at him. Nineteen shots hit Diallo, including one in the bottom of his foot. He was unarmed when he was killed (*Stolen Lives* 1999).

Activists working in communities of color placed police brutality within a larger context of racial and class oppression that turns many people away from direct action. Activists reported that the social and economic conditions of people's lives figured prominently in people's decisions as to whether or not to participate in collective protest. Roberta, a black lesbian, stated that BAM!

> encountered the very real material constraints on people that kept us from doing massive CD [civil disobedience] . . . because we didn't have the same sort of access to people who could get four days off [work]. . . . Some of the people we had were not citizens of the United States. I think we ran into more obstacles that were related to our identity as people of color than ACT UP.

Carlos, a member of ACT UP/New York's Latino Caucus, stated that it was difficult to mobilize people for civil disobedience in a community that is subjected to racist police violence and drug-related arrests on a daily basis. Many white, middle-class, ACT UP activists took for granted being able to be arrested, go to jail, come up with bail money, and get time off from work (Cohen 1998)—issues that were more pressing for working-class and poor people, who are disproportionately people of color.

Furthermore, due to both class and racial biases in the criminal justice system, people of color in general are more likely to have arrest records than white people, and, as a result, are likely to face harsher sentences if arrested during a demonstration. One issue raised by Asian American–Pacific Islander and Latina/o activists was that of legal status. Jeff, a member of the Asian and Pacific Islander Coalition on HIV/AIDS (APICHA) in New York City, commented on the role that immigration status has on direct action participation: "AIDS again is connected to the INS [Immigration and Naturalization Service]. And so people aren't gonna be in droves wanting to get arrested because people could get deported."

Different forms of social inequality shape expectations of elite responses and must be taken into account when analyzing strategies and tactics and political repression. The price of activism weighs more heavily on economically, politically, and socially marginalized groups. Here, it is important to recognize that communities of color are not monolithic with respect to the AIDS crisis. Middle-class activists of any race face less severe consequences for civil disobedience, police brutality, and arrest than poor and working-class activists. Kyle, a black gay man in ACT UP/New York, stated that black middle-class activists typically experience arrest differently than working-class or poor black activists. Patricia, a member of BAM!, stated that her arrest for civil disobedience in New York City while protesting the imprisonment of HIV-positive Haitian refugees at Guantanamo Bay was far more "pleasant" than when she was detained, handcuffed, and harassed by police for an unpaid parking ticket.

Patricia's comments also indicate that the types of tactics used by activists are related to the level of elite repression. The most severe actions taken historically by the FBI and local police forces, such as imprisonment and assassination, have been used against activists (of diverse racial and class backgrounds) who have engaged in armed self-defense or acts of violence targeting the U.S. military-industrial complex, the criminal justice system, and other oppressive systems.[4] Although race and class certainly play a role in shaping both armed struggle and government responses, it is critical to point out that among the more than 100 leftist political prisoners in the United States over the past three decades, a number have been middle-class white women and men (Committee to End the Marion Lockdown 1998).

"Reclaiming" Direct Action

Although expectations of repression—including violence, police abuse, arrest, imprisonment, deportation, and loss of unemployment—are key to understanding the reluctance to engage in direct action, the interviews suggest that the picture is more complex. First, some AIDS activists of color maintained that there is a need to "reclaim" confrontational tactics. Indeed, there were a small number of direct action protests targeting AIDS in communities of color. Second, others contended that although AIDS is a terrible crisis, it is not in and of itself reason enough to warrant engagement in direct action.

Several activists of color in ACT UP expressed frustration with the reluctance of people of color (typically those in other community-based AIDS organizations) to engage in confrontational protest.[5] Several activists stressed that direct action is the only strategy that would produce significant gains. ACT UP/Chicago member Donald stated that "people of color need to understand that ACT UP's tactic was originally *our* [emphasis added] tactic in fighting for African American liberation and so forth, and we need to reclaim it. It's ours." Steven criticized other blacks who were reluctant to take part in the Simi Valley protest against the acquittal of four of the Los Angeles police officers who beat Rodney King:

> I had to remind them that we taught this fucking country how to protest. What's wrong with you people talkin' we don't need to be at Simi Valley? So what if we get our heads bust open. Is that gonna stop us from doin' what we feel is right? . . . Do you think black people got civil rights in this country because we were polite about it? Because we asked for it and we waited patiently until they were ready to give it to us? I don't think so. Black people got their asses kicked, and heads rolled, and people got killed, and people got lynched. And Rosa Parks went to jail, and Martin Luther King was assassinated because we were trying to get a basic civil fucking right! So what makes you think that a disease that is rooted in the community of an ostensibly socially unacceptable—Why do you think this is all gonna happen when George Bush is feeling good one day?

In response to other Puerto Ricans criticizing ACT UP/New York's Latino Caucus for proposing direct action in a general body meeting, Javier stated:

> These people stand up, and they dare to say—to the majority white audience—that what we're proposing is "foreign" to the Latino community, that the Latino community has no knowledge of direct action, it doesn't understand direct action. So we were outraged. . . . If anyone can teach anyone else in this city about direct action, it's the Puerto Rican [community]. . . . Wherever we are now, it's because of people that took over buildings, stopped traffic, or whatever back in the 1960s and 1970s. Where is that legacy? What is happening?

Steven's and Javier's comments reflect two interrelated factors that—along with repression—influenced strategic decisionmaking in communities of color: (1) the perception that direct action is a "white" strategy and (2) the "politics of respectability" that reflect the cooptation of community-based agencies in communities of color (and marginalized communities in general; see Gould 2000; Cohen 1999). Respondents such as Javier expressed dismay that some people of color perceived direct action as a "white thing." Because ACT UP was a primarily white group and because it was the only mass-based AIDS organization using direct action, some activists of color mistakenly classified more confrontational tactics (e.g., civil disobedience) as culturally inappropriate for people of color.

Noel, a staff member at the Asian Pacific AIDS Intervention Team in Los Angeles, stated that there was significant criticism in

communities of color of ACT UP, which he described as "another vehicle for that 1960s type of protest." This comment seems ironic,
given the fact that the model for "1960s type of protest" emerged
within *black* communities during the Civil Rights movement (Morris 1984; McAdam 1982; Carson 1996). Noel described a street theater protest in a predominantly Latino/a neighborhood that received
little support from the community "because they were working on a
Eurocentric model. They were alienating people as opposed to bringing them in." This description suggests that the "problem" might not
have been direct action per se, but the way in which specific actions
are organized and the particular type of direct action taken.

It is clear that the way in which direct action is planned and implemented is extremely important with respect to the social position
(i.e., race, class, gender, sexuality, and other factors) of both participants and targets. But the data also suggest that the denigration of direct action as a whole may be linked to the class privilege of high-
level staff members in mainstream social service agencies serving
communities of color. As discussed in Chapter 2, according to several respondents, those people of color speaking out most vocally
against direct action were often those working for mainstream AIDS
agencies such as the Hispanic AIDS Forum in New York. In Chicago,
Donald asserted that there is a need to do outreach and show people
that they cannot make AIDS go away by being "nice people" and that
gains in the political arena have been made through direct action: "I
don't think [direct action is] a white tactic." Echoing Javier's and
Carlos's critiques of HAF (see Chapter 2), Donald criticized mainstream African American service providers who identified AIDS
protests as a "white thing" but received funding from the government
and worked within the system that caters primarily to white interests.

In the post–Civil Rights movement era, there has been an overall
decline in social protest. It is partly due to the "politics of respectability," that is, the belief that working within the system is the
only legitimate way to work for change. This mindset is in large part
a by-product of the gains (such as the Civil Rights Act of 1964) made
by social movements of the 1960s that led many people in the United
States to believe that there is no longer a need to protest for social
change. There is a plethora of social service agencies serving various
marginalized communities; many of them the products of antiracist
and other forms of political struggle. Although these agencies are
often underfunded and understaffed (and often assimilationist in
ideology), they do provide an illusion that communities are being
adequately "served." The sense of having agencies meeting a commu-

nity's needs helps to reinforce the status quo and the politics of respectability. Furthermore, the administrators who typically run these
organizations are often quite reluctant to jeopardize public and private
funding by participating in or even supporting social protest for more
resources and less discriminatory policies (Stoller 1998). This dynamic
is part of what Donald and Steven referred to when they said that many
AIDS service providers naively think that by being "nice" and "polite," they will be able to adequately challenge the AIDS crisis.

Although many did not engage in direct action AIDS protests
themselves, the vast majority of activists of color viewed direct action,
primarily by ACT UP, as having played a crucial role in the AIDS
movement—including activists critical of ACT UP. Elena stated: "If it
weren't for the direct action of ACT UP, nobody would have AZT [an
anitvirul drug] today." When asked about the role of direct action
AIDS activism, Omar, a gay Latino activist in Los Angeles, stated:

> I think it's been wonderful. I think that without organizations such
> as ACT UP, other organizations like the Life Lobby would not have
> been able to get inside and sit at the table. And I think it's because
> of that kind of demonstration that we have gained more power. And
> it's sad many times where people forget and look down on street
> activism, but basically that's how people react. No one really
> changes or gives up power because they want to give up power. It's
> always because you're fearful of something, and if you see that
> people are rioting, you give in.

In turn, there have been a small number of direct action protests
by groups of people of color. In New York City, BAM! played a key
role in protesting the imprisonment of HIV-positive Haitian refugees
at Guantanamo Bay. This 1993 protest included a picket line at the
Immigration and Naturalization Service's New York office and civil
disobedience leading to arrests. As indicated by Patricia's previous
comments about her arrest, in this situation arrest posed little physical threat to participants. The arrests were worked out ahead of time
with police, who had lists of the arrestees and used plastic handcuffs.[6] Politician Jesse Jackson Sr. and actress Susan Sarandon were
among those arrested. However, even this nonconfrontational action illustrated the differential costs of participation based on class and race.
Participation required spending time away from work and home to attend the protest as well as time in jail, having bail money and legal
representation, and so on—all of which are easier for middle- and
upper-class people of all races (and people who do not have to care

for family members on a daily basis).

In several instances, people of color caucuses within ACT UP executed confrontational protests. On ACT UP's Day of Desperation on January 23, 1991, members of ACT UP/New York's Latino Caucus occupied the office of the Bronx Borough president, while others picketed outside, protesting the lack of city-led action against HIV/AIDS in the Bronx. Maria, against the directive of her boss at Health Force, took several of the Latina women she was training to be AIDS peer educators and participated in the office takeover—as seen in the documentary film *(In)visible Women*. Maria noted that one woman, who later died of AIDS, was transformed by the event and subsequently became active in ACT UP.[7]

Marco, co-founder of Viva, a gay and lesbian Latino/a artist organization in Los Angeles, stated: "We do direct action. That's what we do as artists." As described briefly in Chapter 3, the Divas from Viva utilized *teatro* (street theater) to educate people about HIV/AIDS. In the beginning, these "little guerrilla actions . . . were more political, a lot more illegal." The Divas would close off major Los Angeles streets such as Sunset Boulevard, which initially led to confrontations with the police. Marco also worked with ACT UP/ Los Angeles to put together an informational packet on civil disobedience. In 1990, Viva had a very successful action in which HIV-positive men, trained in civil disobedience, wore chain gang suits and chains, walked about 2 miles and then were arrested by the Los Angeles Police Department. Marco described the direct action tactics during the walk as "wonderful, creative things" such as reading the provocative poem "Howl" by beatnik Allen Ginsberg.

Marco commented that involving parents, children, and other community members helped to turn a protest into a "community action." At one protest, Marco's mother photographed him as he was being arrested. Marco notes that this was effective tactically: "They weren't gonna knock down my mother." Marco stated that it is crucial to design actions "around the people you're working with. . . . If you do that, you're not gonna have any problem with this stuff." Marco remarked that "something that we were trying to deal with was not to be polite as a community." The activism of Viva and other groups presents a challenge to the perspective that direct action protest is "foreign" to communities of color. Such tactics also provide concrete examples of alternative forms of protest carried out despite the possibility of repression.

"A Whole Myriad of Issues"

The interviews also reveal other factors that affected tactical decisions among activists based in communities of color. Several respondents of color articulated the perspective that because there are so many other social problems assaulting communities of color, AIDS in and of itself was not sufficient reason to engage in direct action protest. Many activists were not convinced that AIDS is the most pressing issue facing communities of color, and all agreed that AIDS is intertwined with other social problems. This perspective is related to the discussion in Chapter 3 in which activists of color emphasized that it was crucial to develop strategies that deal more holistically with these issues that are intertwined with HIV/AIDS, particularly on the community level.

Again, this perspective was part of the sometimes unspoken dialogue between the primarily white segments of the movement and people of color. For many gay white men living with HIV/AIDS, the most palpable manifestations of oppression in their lives stemmed from inaction, prejudice, and discrimination related to HIV disease. For people of color, that was not necessarily true. AIDS has been one more injustice to survive and challenge. Jack, a black gay man in BAM!, asserted that people in BAM! thought that ACT UP members "just don't get it. . . . It's not just about AIDS, it's about a whole myriad of other issues." While highlighting other social problems in Native American communities, such as alcoholism, drug addiction, sexism, illiteracy, and other health issues (besides AIDS), Susan, a Native American and Asian American activist in Chicago, stressed: "Talking about AIDS in isolation is a very stupid thing. . . . It's a manipulation of reality."[8]

* * *

Karl Mannheim (1936) believed that human thought processes are shaped by one's position in the social class system. Social location vis-à-vis systems of oppression has a definite impact on the decision to participate in direct action. According to activists of color I interviewed, racial and class oppression continue to be important forces that increase the risk of repression when engaging in social protest and thereby diminish the likelihood of participation in confrontational collective action among people of color, particularly poor and working-class people. Strategic and tactical discussions among activists of color often included an assessment of the potential for police violence and other repercussions. The expectation of repression—police brutality, arrest, imprisonment, deportation, loss of employment—was a factor in tactical discussions assessing the potential for elite violence, in many cases a deterrent factor.

What is particularly important with respect to my data is that knowledge of state efforts to destroy earlier movements continues to promote fear of repression decades later. Along with contemporary racism and classism in the criminal justice system (including police violence), the collective memory of historical repression has had a dampening effect on AIDS activism in communities of color. This temporal dynamic provides a vivid example of how social movement dynamics in one era impact the social movements of another.

Intimidating ACT UP: Cops and Courts

In his cogent examination of historical and contemporary political repression in the United States, Brian Glick shows that government harassment of activists persisted throughout the 1980s, creating "a climate of fear and distrust that undermines our efforts to challenge official policy" (Glick 1989: 5). In this section, I provide evidence supporting Glick's position by analyzing three types of political repression targeting ACT UP during the late 1980s and early 1990s: (1) police abuse; (2) FBI surveillance; and (3) criminal prosecution of ACT UP members.[9] These elite responses drained time, energy, and resources away from fighting AIDS, contributed to burnout, and discouraged people from participating in militant AIDS activism.

As described earlier, ACT UP was a direct action AIDS organization formed in New York City in 1987. The organization used creative, artistic, and confrontational tactics to target government and corporate inaction with regard to AIDS. Although there are still a handful of ACT UP chapters doing key work in the year 2003, most chapters were either nonexistent or extremely deteriorated by the beginning of 1995 (Cohen 1998; Stockdill 2000). Commonly cited factors in the decline of the group include death of members, burnout, cooptation and institutionalization, internal political divisions, reduced press coverage after the early 1990s, and the election of Democrat Bill Clinton in 1992 (Deitcher 1995; Gould 2000).[10] I argue in this section that in addition to these factors (all of which merit more in-depth analysis that is beyond the scope of this book), repression is one frequently overlooked factor in the demise of ACT UP.

As a defiant queer organization, ACT UP's interactions with elites must be placed within the context of a larger system of homophobic oppression. Historically, lesbians, gay men, bisexuals, and transgendered people have been subjected to various forms of abuse from the criminal justice system, particularly police harassment and brutality (Comstock 1991; Deitcher 1995; D'Emilio 1983). Although police brutality, FBI surveillance, and criminal prosecution have also been used historically to repress LGBT activism (Adam 1987), lesbian, gay, and bisexual interview respondents (of all races) in my study did not, by and large, speak about that particular repression. That could be because groups such as the Gay Liberation Front, the Gay Activist Alliance, and various lesbian feminist groups were not targeted with assassinations and draconian prison sentences used to stop groups that employed armed self-defense, such as the Black Panther Party and the American Indian Movement (Churchill and Vander Wall 1990; Committee to End the Marion Lockdown 1998). In my study, white AIDS activists with no prior progressive or radical organizing experience—both inside and outside ACT UP—did not even mention historical repression. In contrast, most people of color as well as white leftists in ACT UP did speak about COINTELPRO and other repressive government campaigns.[11]

Police Abuse

ACT UP/New York member George M. Carter writes that "incidents of police brutality include physical assault and verbal abuse sustained by AIDS activists in Chicago, Philadelphia, New York and elsewhere. This affects AIDS activism directly. The point of AIDS demonstrations is lost in the story of violence while activists continue to face the threat of police brutality" (Carter 1992: 18–19). Interviews with members of ACT UP chapters in New York, Chicago, and Los Angeles revealed numerous instances of police harassment and the use of excessive force at ACT UP demonstrations. In 1990, ACT UP organized a national demonstration in Chicago to call attention to the failures of the U.S. health care system—public and private—and to demand national health insurance. A specific demand of ACT UP/Chicago was that an AIDS ward for women be opened at Cook County Hospital. ACT UP's Women's Caucus created a symbolic AIDS ward by lying down on mattresses, covered with slogans about women and AIDS, in a busy intersection, blocking traffic. Over 100 people were arrested in the demonstration. The AIDS ward was opened the next day. Frank described the protest: "It was a very big, very militant demonstration. It was probably the most militant demonstration that had taken place in Chicago since the 1960s. People were charged by the police on horses. A number of people were seriously injured."

Steven described a sit-in at which ACT UP/Los Angeles members locked themselves to each other around a tree in the atrium of the state of California's Ronald Reagan Building. Their arms were linked together with mountain climbing carabiners and rope inside fiberglass tubes—a tactic used to thwart any attempts to cut them apart. When the police tried to pull their hands apart, the activists explained how they were connected and told the police they would undo themselves. The police kept pulling, however, causing "excruciating pain. . . . That's part of their strategy. . . . They beat the shit out of us and then arrested us."

Steven and most of the other ACT UP respondents reported being subjected to homophobic slurs such as "faggot" and "dyke" by the police in New York, Los Angeles, Chicago, and other cities across the country. Alberto, a Puerto Rican gay man working with VIDA/SIDA, recounted that while a group of ACT UP members were being arrested after a demonstration, the Chicago police were "nasty" and "more physical" with a white gay man "from Radical Fairies [a gay men's organization] wearing a funky dress, cat glasses, and a tasteful wig." The police officers harassed him, saying that "he wasn't a man, he wasn't a woman, he wasn't a human being." The fact that the police singled out for ridicule a protester boldly defying heterosexist norms illustrates the homophobia I observed frequently in my own participation at ACT UP protests.

One other notable aspect of police behavior at ACT UP demonstrations across the nation was the use of plastic gloves. The gloves—which serve no practical purpose in protecting police officers from HIV infection while arresting protesters *presumed* to have HIV/AIDS—highlight the tremendous stigma targeting people living with HIV/AIDS and the extreme ignorance on the part of the police and other segments of mainstream society. The gloves reinforce the popular image that people with HIV/AIDS and by association all AIDS activists, whether HIV-positive or not, are diseased, deserving of ostracism and punishment rather than compassion.

The data indicate that, overall, police repression had a deterrent effect on ACT UP's work. The practice of targeting protest leaders reduced the effectiveness of and in some cases even stopped actions. For example, after the city of Chicago refused to put safer sex and clean needle messages on city buses, ACT UP/Chicago members boarded city buses, gave presentations on safer sex, distributed condoms, exited the buses, walked back, and got on another bus. The Chicago police mounted a camera on top of a store near the bus stop, and according to Stephanie, proceeded to arrest "people who were telling other people what to do. . . . It was just like they knew who to go for." Without leaders to direct the action, the remaining activists found it difficult to continue the action and ended up at the police station bailing out their comrades, who had been arrested on the charge of "mob action."

Several ACT UP members stated that police violence intimidated activists. For example, ACT UP members from Chicago and other cities reported that police reaction was particularly severe at a 1991 action targeting the American Medical Association. According to Ed, an ACT UP/Chicago member, the police came up from behind and started beating and arresting protesters. Some of the people arrested were people who had never been to a demonstration before, and many had not planned on doing civil disobedience. Jackie, an activist and ACT UP/Chicago member, recalled the demonstration: "I saw them [the police] abuse Carrie. I was there when they stood on her back." She continued:

> They separated us. They went right through the middle of us with horses and they just started hitting people right in the crowd. I never want to get arrested in Chicago. . . . I'm very afraid of them, and that's their strategy. If I thought everybody was gonna get arrested, maybe I'd overcome my fear, but I'm just very fearful of Chicago police because I've seen what they've done. . . . So their strategy is effective.

Ed commented on the effect of police violence at the AMA demonstration:

> It had a real chilling effect, and ACT UP never did anything like that since then, until World AIDS Day [December 1992]. . . . That [the police brutality] got a lot of publicity. I sort of feel like it was supposed to 'cause it made it clear that nobody could go to an ACT UP demonstration and not feel like they're gonna get arrested. . . . Meeting attendance and interest in demonstrations really fell off after that.

Ken, a member of ACT UP/New York and then BAM!, traveled to Chicago to participate in the 1990 Cook County Hospital action: "I was arrested in Chicago and that was enough to make me say that

I would never do it again." He stated that the scars on his wrists were still painful three years later. After the 1990 Cook County and 1991 AMA demonstrations, ACT UP publicized the incidents of police brutality in hopes of gaining public sympathy. However, Ed argued that such publicity "was a mistake. It drew attention to all the costs of participating with ACT UP."

Other forms of police intimidation were reported. Javier stated that the Latino Caucus of ACT UP/New York experienced harassing phone calls, phone taps, and infiltration. The caucus often planned demonstrations in secret, and when they arrived at the site of the protest, the police would already be there. Carlos noted that, "We were followed by them [New York City police] when we were planning [a large action]." In some instances, police patrols were stationed outside the ACT UP/New York office. At one point, a police officer called Carlos's house and asked him if he knew of any upcoming demonstrations. Other members of ACT UP/New York, ACT UP/Los Angeles, and ACT UP/Chicago reported similar occurrences.

FBI Surveillance

Even though harassment by the FBI and other federal agencies was not as prevalent in the data as police abuse, several activists did speak about this form of social control. Most ACT UP members in the study were aware that FBI files released under the Freedom of Information Act show that ACT UP was the subject of "domestic terrorism" and "civil unrest" investigations since its birth in 1987 (Carter 1992; Wolfe 1993). A campaign of harassing phone calls and death threats that targeted ACT UP women nationally in the early 1990s is speculated by ACT UP members to be a part of the FBI's harassment of ACT UP. Maria stated that "the police do not act alone. . . . The U.S. and other capitalist nations actively organize to stop any potential radical organizing that might lead to revolutionary movements." According to Maria, as part of this repressive strategy, antiterrorist forces were sent to ACT UP protests dressed as regular police. This activity should be seen within the context of wider repressive efforts taken by the U.S. government at different levels. For example, Ward Churchill and Jim Vander Wall (1990; see also Glick 1989) documented "FBI police amalgams," joint FBI–local police units, used to suppress political dissidence in New York City and other U.S. cities in the 1980s. More recently, local police forces and other government authorities have infiltrated progressive and radical organizations and attended rallies disguised as "protesters" in order to gather information and repress antiglobalization and other activists. The police have beaten, shot, and arrested activists (and journalists) at demonstrations in Los Angeles; Seattle; Washington, D.C.; and Genoa, Italy, where one protester was killed.

Echoing the work of Gary Marx (1974), Ruud Koopmans concludes in an article on protest waves in West Germany: "The repression and marginalization of these [radical] groups also stimulates sectarian conflicts and distrust among activists, which diverts energy from external activities and discourages outsiders from participating" (Koopmans 1993: 655). The testimonies of AIDS activists support Koopmans's argument. Experiences with the police and the FBI as well as knowledge of past COINTELPRO activities among leftist members promoted fear and mistrust in many ACT UP chapters. At the beginning of every ACT UP/Chicago general body meeting, police officers and journalists were asked to identify themselves and leave. New members were sometimes suspected of being police informants. Fearful that committee members' apartments might be bugged, members of ACT UP/Chicago's Prison Issues Committee established the practice of writing down protest times and dates rather than saying them out loud.[12]

Criminal Prosecution

The third form of repression that targeted ACT UP is the criminal prosecution of ACT UP members. Across the nation, ACT UP members were arrested, spent time in jail, and in some cases faced lengthy and costly legal battles. In one instance, multiple felony charges were filed against the Houston Three (members of ACT UP/New York) for their participation at a protest at the 1992 Republican Party Convention in Houston, Texas (Wolfe 1993). One particular case involving the prosecution of three ACT UP/Denver members provides a striking example of homophobic repression.[13]

On January 14, 1993, AIDS activists draped plastic bags bearing the word *AIDS* over tombstones in a Catholic cemetery in Jefferson County, Colorado—to dramatize the Catholic Church's complicity in the AIDS crisis by its condemnation of homosexuality and condom use (an effective means of preventing HIV transmission).[14] In the spring of 1993, three ACT UP/Denver members moved out of Colorado (to Los Angeles and Chicago), in large part to escape the violently homophobic political climate that surrounded the passage of Amendment 2, an amendment to the Colorado constitution (later overturned by the U.S. Supreme Court) that prohibited civil rights protection for lesbians and gay men and, in effect, legalized discrimination and promoted violence against LGBT individuals and groups.

Despite the fact that an initial investigation in January 1993 was dropped due to lack of evidence, a grand jury was convened and indictments against the three ACT UP/Denver members were issued on August 12, 1993—the eve of the pope's and then President Clinton's arrival for a visit to Denver. The state of Colorado launched an aggressive prosecution, filing two felony charges and two misdemeanor charges carrying possible sentences of twenty-six years—certainly excessive for a vandalism case. The Catholic Church, which had worked arduously to win the passage of Amendment 2, vigorously demanded the prosecution of the activists. All three activists spent at least a week in jail and were interrogated by law enforcement officers without their lawyers being present. Courtney, a white lesbian, was held in Los Angeles and transported in a van to Colorado and placed in jail. Thomas and John, both HIV-positive white gay men, were interrogated by U.S. Secret Service agents and thrown into Cook County Jail in Chicago, where guards announced to other inmates that they were "faggots with AIDS" and "pope-killers." Thomas and John were subsequently extradited to Colorado. Their T-cell counts dropped precipitously by over 500 (normal T-cell counts range between 800 and 1,200) during the months following their arrest.

Historically, grand juries have been used by the government as a tool to divide and conquer social movements such as the Catholic left, the Puerto Rican independence movement, the American Indian Movement, the women's movement, and the movement to end the Vietnam War (Churchill and Vander Wall 1990; Glick 1989). Grand jury proceedings are secret, and people who refuse to testify can be thrown in jail for contempt. Activists and others are often interrogated about organizations, demonstrations, civil disobedience, and so on. According to ACT UP/Chicago's Legal Defense Committee literature: "A grand jury was used to divide the lesbian, gay, and AIDS activist movement in Colorado. The state's attorney was able to intimidate members of the lesbian and gay community and gather testimony pointing fingers at radical activists to produce indictments against the three ACT UP members." Twenty out of forty-six grand jury witnesses were reportedly lesbians and gay men, and the other twenty-six were police officers. One former member of ACT UP/Denver initially implicated in the action testified against the defendants—reportedly after the state threatened to take custody of her child.

At least one police officer alleged that the defendants were conspiring against the pope—despite the fact that all three were out of the state for several months before the indictments. Legal Defense Committee literature states their framing of the events: "The fact that the indictments and arrests occurred simultaneously with the arrival of the Pope and the President in Denver reveals Colorado's absurd attempt to paint those indicted as dangerous people who posed a threat to the Pope and the President."

The severity of the charges, the allegations of a conspiracy against the pope, the political climate fostered by Amendment 2, and the use of a grand jury supports ACT UP's claim that the Denver case represents the criminalization of queer and AIDS activism. The Legal Defense Committee writes that the activists were targeted in order to "punish them for their activism and discourage others from vocally opposing the Catholic Church's policies and fighting the AIDS crisis with direct action protest. . . . The members of ACT UP/Denver were targeted not for putting plastic bags on tombstones, but for being outspoken, queer AIDS activists."

The Denver case had a debilitating effect on ACT UP. On a financial level, tens of thousands of dollars had to be raised for bail and the defense campaign—most of it by ACT UP/Chicago and other ACT UPs across the nation. Perhaps more significant was the intimidation of AIDS and queer activists in Denver. According to Legal Defense Committee member Jennifer, a white lesbian, "The homophobic hysteria that fueled Amendment 2 had already led the three activists to move from Denver to Los Angeles and Chicago. The grand jury had the effect of intimidating and dividing Denver activists, decimating what was left of ACT UP/Denver."

ACT UP/Denver fell apart after these events. The case sowed bitter conflict between different activists and organizations in the Denver gay and lesbian community. Some activists in Denver lashed out against the indicted ACT UP members. Jennifer stated: "The grand jury caught people off guard. The movement was quickly swept up in vicious arguments about ACT UP's tactics, the cemetery action and so on, rather than the despicable actions taken by the state." In the long run, ACT UP members—inside and outside Denver—felt that the case served to weaken the movement by once again revealing the potential costs of direct action AIDS activism.[15]

* * *

Koopmans asserts: "The interplay between facilitation, repression, and the chance of success defines a set of external constraints that combine with activists' choices among three strategic options—innovation, increased participation, or increased militancy" (Koopmans 1993: 637). In the case of ACT UP, facilitation can be seen as government and corporate support for the burgeoning AIDS industry that employs tens of thousands of people across the country. Many activists have traded in militancy for paid positions in mainstream AIDS agencies. This flight from the movement was reinforced by government repression, particularly for those faced with the threat of dying with AIDS.

Although many HIV-positive activists joined ACT UP to fight for their very lives, the stress of living with HIV served as a weapon that heightened the costs of AIDS activism. When contemplating the consequences of participation, many AIDS activists had to assess the impact participation would have on their health.[16] Emotional and physical burnout took a significant toll on those not infected with HIV as well. Several respondents reported that it was difficult to continue their activism after watching so many of their comrades get sick and die. It is hard to sustain a movement in the midst of such widespread illness and death. Fear of police brutality, FBI surveillance, and prosecution coupled with a compromised immune system and burnout undoubtedly discouraged confrontational activism. In turn, it appears that the remains of ACT UP failed to muster the innovation or militancy that might have provided the spark needed to breathe life into the organization in the mid-1990s.

The Impact of Repression

Given the extensive documentation of political repression in the United States, the lack of attention given to repression in social movement literature is troubling, to say the least.[17] Robert White and Terry White note that when analyses of state repression are presented there is "a tendency . . . to focus on repression in non-democratic and non-Western states" (White and White 1994: i). Aside from the problematic assumptions frequently made as to what exactly constitutes a "democratic" or "Western" state, this observation is a keen one. For example, Karl-Dieter Opp and Christiane Gern write: "In authoritarian regimes, an expectation of repression is a central variable explaining participation in protests" (Opp and Gern 1993: 661), but in "Western democracies," "communication critical of the incumbent government or political system can be exchanged without fear of severe repression" (1993: 659).

Such misleading assumptions about "authoritarian" versus "democratic" governments held by social movement scholars prevent meaningful sociological analysis of the role played by repression in the development of social movements in the United States and other ostensibly democratic countries. If sociologists studying social movements challenged such assumptions, there could be more useful research on COINTELPRO and other government-sponsored attempts to crush leftist collective action—research that could optimally provide a wealth of information for social movement theory.

Within "democratic" countries, there is a need to examine the protesters' relationship to existing systems of domination. The data for my study demonstrate that systems of racial, class, and homophobic inequality are intertwined with potential participants' expectations and actual experiences of repression.[18] Government attacks on social movements shape tactical and strategic choices within the context of systemic marginalization. Fear of repression—especially police brutality and imprisonment—makes political organizing around AIDS especially difficult for those activists who advocate direct action.

The findings clearly illustrate the importance of the social position of social movement participants with respect to political repression.[19] As detailed by Cohen (1999), the complex marginalization of black communities has shaped African Americans' collective responses to the AIDS crisis. The evidence in my study indicates that within communities of color, the expectation of repression—rooted in collective memory and present-day experiences—is another key factor influencing AIDS activism in black and other communities of color. Familiarity with widespread racist police abuse and racial and class bias in the judicial system dimmed the prospects of confrontational political struggle—though some activists of color have continued to advocate militant social protest. Outside the arena of AIDS, activists engaged in direct action tactics throughout the 1990s and made significant gains. For example, janitors participating in Justice for Janitors campaigns, many of them undocumented workers from Mexico and El Salvador, have protested for (and in some cases won) a living wage, health insurance, improved working conditions, and the right to unionize. In many cases, these activists faced police brutality, arrests, termination of employment, and deportation.

Decisions on whether to participate in AIDS direct action were shaped not only by contemporary threats of coercion but by collective memories of past repression of social movements. The finding that elite repression from one era stretches across decades to instill fear among activists in another era adds another dimension to McAdam's (1983) concept of tactical interaction. The tactical responses embodied in the FBI's COINTELPRO activities were not only critical in the demise of radical movements in the 1960s and 1970s, but their social psychological imprint also impeded radical AIDS organizing in the 1980s and 1990s. AIDS activists—in communities of color and in ACT UP—experienced extreme difficulty developing new tactics to overcome fear and effectively counter government repression.

Most members of ACT UP, a primarily middle-class, white organization, had a different relationship to racial and class systems of oppression. Most middle-class white ACT UP members did not initially have a collective perception that they would be brutalized by the police or the FBI or both, nor did they anticipate spending decades in prison as a result of their activism. Thus, many felt less threatened participating in direct action than activists of color. ACT UP also typically had access to more financial, political, and social resources than many organizations of color (Stoller 1998; Cohen 1998). For these reasons, they were better positioned to deal with arrests and criminal charges than activists working in communities of color.

However, white skin and middle-class privileges do not prevent repression. As queers using often militant and disruptive tactics, ACT UP members were subjected to homophobic sanctions. Though certainly not as severe as the COINTELPRO violence of the 1960s and 1970s, local, state, and federal authorities brought to bear considerable resources to undermine the only nationwide, direct action organization fighting AIDS—ACT UP. Police harassment and abuse intimidated activists and discouraged potential activists from becoming involved in ACT UP. FBI surveillance added to the fear of government assault and fomented mistrust within many ACT UP chapters. The prosecution of activists drained away valuable time, energy, and financial resources. The stress and uncertainty facing HIV-positive ACT UP members raised the stakes of taking part in social protest. Though clearly not the only factor, the data demonstrate that repression weakened the group and played a role in its demise.

Despite criticisms of racism and sexism in the organization, most chapters consistently formed groups—particularly caucuses organized by women and people of color—that sought to embrace a broader and more radical set of political concerns. George Carter, of ACT UP/New York, implicitly links repression to ACT UP's movement to the left: "As ACT UP broadens its base to be more inclusive of different views and people in true coalition, there is the potential for broad-based, radical change that threatens the inimical power base of both government and the giant pharmaceutical industry" (Carter 1992: 19). This increasing radicalism was seen in ACT UP's efforts in the areas of housing, clean needle exchanges, prisoners' rights, sex workers' rights, political prisoners, and opposition to the U.S. war on Iraq in 1991, as well as coalitions with health care workers, the Puerto Rican independence movement, and environmental, labor, and other groups. It is precisely in these areas where people of color, women, and other marginalized groups worked with ACT UP, but such efforts were thwarted by the deterioration of the organization.

In conclusion, the data suggest that the combined weight of actual repression targeting ACT UP and expected repression among many activists of color operated to inhibit coalitions between different communities and organizations and to reinforce racial and class rifts in the AIDS movement. More research on the AIDS movement and other movements is needed to test this theory. Such research will hopefully help us more fully understand the relationship between intersecting oppressions, consciousness, strategies, and repression. The finding that collective memories of historic state repression have left an imprint on collective consciousness is an important start. In turn, activists must develop innovative protest methods to confront government repression and push forward radical campaigns for social change.

6

Conclusion: An Intersectional Approach to Social Movement Research and Activism

> Having been an activist in different areas, I believe that holistic approaches are key, approaches that make connections between different oppressions. It's so important to understand that racism affects immigration experiences, it affects domestic violence, it affects HIV/AIDS. Sexism has a role in education, in poverty. Homophobia hurts gay immigrants and youth. A holistic vision that will help people understand and take action is essential in achieving social justice.
>
> —Catalina, AIDS caseworker, Detroit

Throughout this book, I have examined some of the ways in which multiple oppressions influence collective action. Examining AIDS activism from different angles of vision demonstrates the importance of developing more inclusive and intersectional approaches to both social movement theory and activism. Just as interlocking inequalities have shaped the epidemiology of the disease, they have affected the collective battles waged against AIDS. At every step, activism has been complicated by multiple systems of oppression. Internal movement conflict, activist strategies, and elite repression have been intertwined with heterosexual, gender, racial, and class domination.

An intersectional framework sheds light on the links between the structural, cultural, and personal levels of social movement development. Theoretical approaches attentive to the interactions of multiple inequalities provide finer tools with which to investigate social movements. Below, I outline five theoretical propositions that illuminate how intersectionality shapes the landscape of social movement activity. I then discuss the implications of these propositions for social movement scholarship as well as activism.

Social Movement Theory, AIDS Activism, and Intersectionality

As discussed in Chapters 1–5, the breadth and depth of social movement activity is not adequately addressed by resource mobilization models and social psychological approaches. Social movement scholars in both camps have typically examined social movements within the context of one particular system of oppression and have failed to look at how other inequalities affect collective action. Thus, they have not unveiled the vulnerability of social movements to multiple systems of domination or the formulation of collective endeavors to breach this vulnerability and build more radical, inclusive political coalitions.

Analysis of the AIDS movement vividly illustrates Carol Mueller's (1992) perspective that social movement participants are "socially embedded." The social location of individual activists shapes their experiences and identities. Social location with respect to systematic inequalities impacts the consciousness, culture, organizations, resources, and strategies of communities engaging in protest. My analysis of the AIDS movement shows that collective action is mediated by an individual or organization's social location in relation to *multiple* social hierarchies.

The matrix of race, class, gender, and heterosexual oppressions creates a complex set of conditions for social movements. Five theoretical propositions related to the effect of multiple oppressions on collective action can be drawn from analysis of the AIDS movement.

1. *Partial oppositional consciousness emanating from multiple systems of oppression often results in internal movement conflict.* As described in Chapter 1, members of oppressed groups—LGBTs, injection drug users, people of color, poor people, prisoners (and, in particular, those in two or more of these groups, such as African American and Latino gay men)—have been disproportionately hit by HIV/AIDS. Dominant society's response to the epidemic has been shaped by stigma and institutional bigotry. What is less clear to the

outside observer is the extension of various forms of oppression into communities affected by AIDS and into the AIDS movement itself. In contrast to mainstream resource mobilization and social psychological approaches, my intersectional analysis reveals the fissures created by the differential social locations and consciousnesses of participants and movement organizations. These fissures have sapped the time and energy of activists in many different AIDS organizations and inhibited the formation of coalitions necessary to sustain a more unified, broad-based movement.

As presented in Chapter 2, conflicting ideological frames emerged within the AIDS movement, leading to internal movement conflict. These ideological frames were frequently linked to participants' locations in multiple social hierarchies. Within the direct action group ACT UP, for example, two ideological perspectives often clashed. The first perspective, which embodies partial oppositional consciousness, framed AIDS as a discrete social problem unrelated to sexism, classism, and racism. This ideological stance was typically, though not exclusively, held by middle-class white gay men with little prior activist experience. This group faces homophobic oppression and frequently related AIDSphobia but generally benefits from racial, class, and gender privilege. Their oppositional consciousness often centered on homophobia/AIDSphobia to the exclusion of other forms of domination. As a result, strategies flowing from this consciousness often focused on a search for a cure to HIV/AIDS, access to clinical drug trials, speedier government approval of promising treatments, reduction of the cost of antiviral medications, and other related issues. These strategies led to very important gains in the areas of AIDS research and treatment, but the lack of a genuine understanding of or commitment to how these and other issues affect poor people, people of color, and women meant that access to health care and fulfillment of other needs remained skewed along gender, racial, and class lines.

The second perspective within ACT UP viewed AIDS as intertwined with not only homophobia but racism, sexism, and classism—a perspective used for social action articulated since the 1970s by feminists of color and lesbian feminists (particularly lesbians of color). This ideological position was typically held by ACT UP members who were people of color and women, particularly those who had prior activist experience. These participants—and the communities in which they were embedded—faced not only homophobia/AIDSphobia but racism, classism, and/or sexism. This oppositional consciousness was multidimensional, taking aim at not one but several forms of domination. As I stated in Chapter 2, it would be inaccurate to say that these activists and organizations attained some "ultimate" oppositional consciousness that is completely inclusive of all inequalities. Rather, they were attentive to the social groups that are often neglected by more mainstream activism, and this attentiveness includes active discussions and actions at the intersections of oppressions. Within the context of AIDS activism, such groups called for broader, more inclusive strategies that emphasize the impact of AIDS on injection drug users, prisoners, women, people of color, and the poor. Examples of specific campaigns created by these activists are community-based clean needle exchanges and AIDS in prison projects.

Much time and energy was given to heated debates over the two approaches to AIDS activism in many ACT UP chapters. In some cities, ACT UP chapters split into separate groups over such conflicts. As seen in Chapter 2, there are other examples of competing political consciousnesses within movement organizations, such as gender conflicts within BAM! and class conflicts within ACT UP/ New York's Latino Caucus. In other instances, there have been organizational conflicts in which smaller community-based organizations (e.g., the AIDS Prevention Team) criticized "mega-agencies" (e.g., the AIDS Project Los Angeles) for not providing adequate services for women, poor people, and people of color.

In general, partial oppositional consciousness within a social movement with diverse participants and organizations is likely to result in internal divisions. Activists and organizations targeting a single oppression are also likely to have one or more connections to sites of power and privilege that blind them to the ways in which they actually reinforce other forms of oppression. As a consequence, movement participants and organizations concerned with multiple oppressions are forced to fight for more inclusive strategies, tactics, and resources. This conflict reduced the overall effectiveness of the AIDS movement.

On the community level, partial oppositional consciousness presented a stumbling block for AIDS activists fighting AIDS among women, people of color, injection drug users, and prisoners. For example, activists had to challenge homophobia within communities of color in order to gain the support of established political, social, and religious organizations. Homophobic consciousness among Asian American, Latino/a, and black heterosexual leaders and organizations often resulted in inaction regarding the AIDS epidemic. Homophobic consciousness within communities of color has often been manifested in a compartmentalization of race and sexuality that views being gay and of color as mutually exclusive. This dichotomy results in a situation in which strongly identifying with one's racial community and thus being "antiracist" often requires one to be homophobic. On a concrete level, particularly during the early years of the epidemic, this conflict often led to a head-in-the-sand approach to AIDS: "Only gay people get AIDS, and people of color aren't gay, so there's no problem in our community." This example shows how partial oppositional consciousness prevents community unity and consequently inhibits mobilization of a more unified front capable of making demands on dominant social institutions, such as the federal government and the medical establishment. It also shows how denial can be deadly.

One pattern evident throughout the data is the difficulty participants had in dealing with class issues. Class divisions within communities of color have created "access" problems for middle-class activists. Their middle-class status has sometimes resulted in social distancing from working-class and poor communities. Several members of BAM!, for example, stated that more genuine dialogues about class were needed to build bridges within the African American communities. According to several respondents, many progressive activists tend to pay more attention to race, gender, and sexuality than class. Class seems to be less tangible, more difficult to identify, and—perhaps—more sensitive and even painful as a subject of self-reflection. That could be because AIDS activists developing strategies and tactics have been disproportionately middle class and are blind to their own privilege, reluctant to discuss class privilege openly and critically, or simply overwhelmingly frustrated to the point of inaction. According to members of ACT UP/New York's Latino Caucus, the Hispanic AIDS Forum was oblivious to its own class privilege and consequently did not fulfill its mission to provide HIV/AIDS services to Hispanics in New York.

When it comes to discussing white people and the AIDS epidemic, class is often obscured. Among many activists—both white people and people of color—class is often discussed in relationship to African Americans and other people of color, but this is less true in relationship to whites, the underlying false assumption being that the vast majority of white people are middle or upper class. Only two respondents (interestingly, working-class African Americans) brought up the issue of poor and working-class whites within the context of the AIDS crisis, stating that this population is frequently left out of prevention and intervention strategies. In this situation, race (being white) is generally perceived as the defining characteristic, despite the fact that class (being poor or working class) may be a more important factor influencing one's health status. People's position within a racial hierarchy was seen as the main factor that determines their relationship to AIDS, and class was not a primary consideration. This neglect of class issues reflects the lack of critical attention given to working-class and poor whites by both social scientists and many activists of all races.

Theoretically, partial oppositional consciousness provides a conceptual bridge linking systems of oppression, social movement actors and organizations, and collective action strategies. The social location of social movement participants and potential participants is associated with their political consciousness. Gay white men are located in a subordinate position relative to heterosexual oppression but benefit from racial and gender privilege. Thus, they tend to have a consciousness that opposes homophobia but reinforces racial and gender oppression, whether intentionally or not. Heterosexual men of color, in turn, often display antiracist consciousness but have positions of power and privilege with respect to sexism and homophobia. These political consciousnesses often lead to strategies that challenge only one form of domination. Consequently, "community" boundaries are drawn that exclude lesbians and gay men of color. Interlocking systems of oppression survive intact.

As discussed in Chapter 2, analysis of partial oppositional consciousness within the AIDS movement provides clear evidence that multiple systems of oppression are interlocking—a key component of black feminist theory (and the more recently articulated "multiracial feminist theory"). Human systems of domination are replicated within oppressed populations, creating a crisscrossing set of chains shackling communities in subordination and marginalization. Breaking one chain is insufficient to gain full freedom because another chain continues to bind.

In addition, the data indicate that these oppressions often operate simultaneously, as seen in the case of prisoners, gay and bisexual men of color, and women of color living with HIV/AIDS. This finding calls into question efforts to prioritize inequalities that reflect traditional conceptualizations of systems of inequality as discrete rather than interactive. For example, narrow racial nationalism downplays or even promotes homophobia and sexism, and mainstream LGBT activism often ignores racism, classism, and sexism. The simultaneity of intersecting inequalities explored in this book provides support for interactive models of social stratification (King 1988; Collins 1990; Smith 1983).

2. *Multiple systems of inequality promote an unequal distribution of resources among disparate movement sectors and prevent low-resource segments from tapping into established resource pools.* In terms of the AIDS movement's relationship to dominant society, it is clear that multiple systems of domination have restricted access to resources necessary to fight the disease (see Stoller 1998). Homophobic consciousness translated into genocidal neglect, particularly during the 1980s. A central task of AIDS activists has been to challenge homophobia and the devaluation of queer lives on a societal level to build public support for establishing and increasing federal, state, and municipal AIDS funding.

Homophobia, however, has not been the only form of oppression entrenched in the AIDS crisis. Even as gay and lesbian communities forced the government and other institutions to take action, gender, race, and class-biased public policies have diminished the availability of financial and other resources for AIDS programs for other severely affected communities, frequently compounding the impact of homophobia. In an era of political conservatism marked by cuts in social service programs for the poor, AIDS activists have faced increasingly difficult battles obtaining funds for marginalized populations such as poor women of color, prisoners, and addicts. These and other groups continue to be hit hard from different directions in 2003. For example, poor women of color face significant difficulties obtaining welfare benefits, housing, child care, and food subsidies, as well as educational and employment opportunities. This precarious situation—produced by the systemic assaults of racism, sexism, and classism—increases their vulnerability to HIV infection. For those already infected with HIV, these threats increase the probability of a quickened descent into full-blown AIDS.

The predicament of prisoners provides another illustration of the effect of multiple oppressions on the accessibility of resources. As demonstrated in Chapter 4, homophobic, racial, and class inequalities (and sexism for female prisoners) have created a situation in which prisoners are not only denied quality AIDS care but also are deprived of the resources necessary to engage in collective action to demand better HIV/AIDS-related services. The conditions of isolation and dehumanization accompanying incarceration restrict access to various resources, thereby inhibiting protest.

On the community and movement levels, partial oppositional consciousness robs smaller movement organizations—particularly those outside the middle- and upper-class, white, gay male sphere—of important resources. Financially and politically connected AIDS mega-agencies such as Gay Men's Health Crisis in New York City have been able to raise millions of dollars in single fund-raising events, but race, class, and gender inequities often prevented these funds from reaching small, community-based organizations providing services to people of color, the poor, and women. As discussed in Chapter 2, respondents working in small, community-based organizations providing services to women and people of color reported that primarily white, middle-class mega-agencies tended to hog scarce funds while failing to establish accessible and culturally sensitive programs for other populations. Although significant gains have been made in recent years in this area, inequity is still a problem in the AIDS "industry." Similarly, as seen in Chapter 4, prison AIDS activists face an uphill battle in obtaining the support of mainstream AIDS agencies, in large part as a result of an ideology that perceives the lives of prisoners as less important than others. Unfortunately, the outlook for prisoners with HIV/AIDS remains grim in the first decade of the twenty-first century.

Mainstream AIDS agencies in the gay community have not been the only organizations accused of not sharing resources (and compassion) in the fight against AIDS. Homophobia in communities of color has made it difficult for AIDS activists to gain the support of various institutions and organizations in Asian, African American, and Latino/a communities. For example, homophobia has often prevented African American AIDS activists from tapping into the rich organizational potential of the African American church—a key institution in historical social movements such as the Civil Rights movement. In recent years, some African American churches, and churches in general, have begun to rethink bigoted positions on homosexuality, but the bulk (of churches, synagogues, and mosques) have yet to fully accept and welcome their LGBT members, even as AIDS continues to kill.

In general, the lack of resources available to fight AIDS and the skewed distribution of existing resources is directly related to partial oppositional consciousness. A more inclusive oppositional consciousness would facilitate more equal access to resources, which in turn would enable previously separate groups to coalesce and demand increased resources from the government and other institutions. There are several cases in the data of different groups working together to maximize their resource pools. In Los Angeles in the early 1990s, the Asian Pacific AIDS Intervention Team, the Minority AIDS Project, Bienestar, Teatro Viva, and the AIDS Prevention Team found themselves shut out of the funding game and fighting over the crumbs left by AIDS Project Los Angeles. They formed a consortium and were collectively able to secure a significantly higher level of outside funding. Outside AIDS activists have been crucial in developing collective action efforts to combat AIDS in prison. These AIDS activists work in solidarity with prisoners to improve educational programs, access to the means of prevention, and various services to prisoners with HIV/AIDS. Prisoners have provided the documentation necessary to expose the dramatic flaws in prison AIDS programs and have assessed their specific HIV/AIDS-related needs. Prison AIDS activists outside the prison wall often have access to certain resources, based on both class privilege and links to various social movement communities. These connections have helped in publicizing the problem of AIDS in prison, gaining support from other groups, and pushing for change.

    3. *Multiple inequalities increase radical movement sectors' vulnerability to repression, dividing the broader movement and undermining the potential benefits of a united front.* As shown in Chapter 5, the combined weight of expected and actual repression weakened the AIDS movement, reducing its potential to bring about change. This repression is rooted in multiple systems of domination. This *repression effect* has implications for other contemporary movements and may help explain the relatively low prevalence of militant, confrontational strategies and tactics.

    Activists of color reported that knowledge of the FBI's repression of radical 1960s' antiracist groups, particularly the Black Panther Party, had a stifling effect on contemporary social protest. Knowledge of past government repression, including surveillance, murder, and imprisonment, discouraged the use of more confrontational methods of protest. Collective memories of repression illuminate the links between social structure, consciousness, and collective action. The historical use of violence by the U.S. government to crush movements for racial equality is etched upon the minds of many contemporary activists of color—potentially sources of militant political activism. Fear of similar reprisals (and other factors discussed in Chapter 3) shaped the formulation of strategies and tactics to fight AIDS and resulted in less confrontational approaches that have been less likely to demand fundamental restructuring of the health care system and other social systems.

Collective memories of the FBI's COINTELPRO unit were compounded by contemporary perceptions of racial and class bias on the part of the police and within the criminal justice system. Black and Latino/a activists were (and are) well aware of the epidemic of racially motivated police brutality and the swelling prison population throughout the 1990s, which is disproportionately composed of poor and working-class people of color. The contemporary threat of violence and imprisonment presented by the criminal justice system worked as another inhibiting force on the AIDS movement.

ACT UP, which boldly confronted homophobia, AIDSphobia, and other forms of inequality, faced police brutality, FBI surveillance, and criminal prosecution. At its most radical points, ACT UP worked to expose how the devastation caused by the AIDS epidemic has been fueled by systematic oppression. In doing so, the organization moved beyond more moderate movement organizations that have typically worked within the system rather than challenging it. ACT UP's militant politic was met with negative sanctions from the mass media, the police, and the government. The harsh treatment of ACT UP parallels the treatment of the radical sectors of other movements. Analysis of the AIDS movement demonstrates that radical sectors of social movements—those that most vociferously work to expose and change structural inequities—are most likely to face repression from elites. This situation encouraged other segments of the movement to distance themselves from ACT UP—a pattern evident in many of the interviews as well as my participant observation—and served to reduce the possibility of coalition building across the AIDS movement.

In addition, the stigma, fear, and stress of living with HIV operated as natural weapons of repression—undoubtedly preventing many from participating in collective action in the years before protease inhibitors were widely available (1995–1996) and causing burnout among movement participants living with HIV/AIDS. The costs of militant AIDS activism—violence, arrest, jail time—were significantly higher for people living with HIV/AIDS.

The dynamics of repression further show the importance of analyzing the links between multiple oppressions and social movement development. These dynamics, as related to the AIDS movement, have emanated from homophobic, sexist, racist, and classist systems of domination. Overall, attacking the most radical, mass-based sector of the AIDS movement—ACT UP—had a dampening effect. The targeting of ACT UP by the FBI, police, and courts was one important factor in the decline of street-level AIDS protest in the mid-1990s.

More moderate AIDS groups were even more likely to be intimidated and even less likely to engage in direct action protest.

Past repression of antiracist and anti-imperialist movements and organizations (such as the Puerto Rican independence movement) served to diminish the prospects of more militant AIDS activism in communities of color. This finding undoubtedly has implications for other forms of collective action in communities of color. It seems logical that collective memories of COINTELPRO, along with familiarity with racist police violence, serve to reduce the potential for radical political struggle used to remedy other social problems such as unemployment, racial and class biases in the criminal justice system, environmental racism, and urban education, particularly within the context of class divisions in communities of color.

Repression affects not only the actions of individual organizations but the relationships between these organizations. Although other AIDS groups have sometimes rallied behind ACT UP in the face of government attacks, it appears that, in many cases, they have tried to distance themselves from the direct action group. The fear of racist police brutality and imprisonment, coupled with many white activists' ignorance of this racist repression, also led some people of color to be reluctant to participate in or ally themselves with ACT UP. Thus, the potential benefits of unity have been thwarted by the complex dynamics related to actual and expected repression. These dynamics exist in other areas of collective action as well (e.g., racial and class rifts in the environmental justice movement).

4. *The existence of interlocking inequalities on different levels (personal, institutional, cultural) necessitates collective action that targets not only dominant institutions but also individuals, marginalized communities, and movement organizations.* Resource mobilization models have typically focused on social movement activity targeting dominant social institutions. An analytical framework attentive to intersecting inequalities reveals the broader scope of collective action, particularly the important role of challenging hegemonic ideology.

As seen throughout the book, AIDS activism clearly shows the usefulness of social psychological models that highlight the transformation of collective consciousness as a key aspect of the mobilization process. Indeed, a central aspect of AIDS organizing has been challenging dominant norms around homosexuality (and sexuality in general), drug addiction, prisoners, and health care. Analysis of the AIDS movement provides support for Snow and his colleagues' 1986 theory of frame alignment, according to which activists rely on "micromobilization" strategies to realign the ideological views of potential participants. However, the concept of frame alignment theory does little to illuminate the interaction of multiple forms of political consciousnesses during the micromobilization process.

As described in Chapter 2, partial oppositional consciousness creates the need to address inequalities on the community and movement levels. Movements that primarily target only one form of inequality (the Civil Rights movement) are more likely to focus social change efforts on changing dominant social institutions (e.g., state and federal legal systems) and realigning one stream of political consciousness (e.g., racist ideology) within dominant society. However, in the case of the AIDS crisis, which is more visibly driven by multiple oppressions, community-level inequalities have been paramount. Because marginalized communities are fractured internally by systems of oppression, activists challenging multiple forms of inequality, as seen in Chapters 3 and 4, must work within communities to foster a broader oppositional consciousness. Thus, women in communities of color have worked to fight sexist gender roles that increase women's risk of HIV infection. Lesbians and gay men of color have made significant gains in combating homophobic collective beliefs within Asian American, black, and Latino/a communities.

This collective action occurs not only within the community but also within movement organizations themselves. Social movement organizations are not immune to partial oppositional consciousness. Women's caucuses in ACT UP consistently attempted to integrate not only feminism but antiracist and leftist politics into the group's strategies. Sometimes partial oppositional consciousness prevailed, resulting in organizational splits, defections, and burnout. However, in other instances, group ideologies and strategies were transformed to be more inclusive in challenging multiple forms of domination, such as a focus on improved treatment access for women and people of color.[1]

As seen in Chapter 4, prison AIDS activists found that relying on instrumental strategies was insufficient to bring about change. In response, they created campaigns targeting both mainstream AIDS agencies and Chicago's North Side LGBT community to humanize prisoners and garner support for AIDS in prison activism but achieved mixed results. Across the country, the resources available to prisoners and former prisoners with HIV/AIDS have increased, but there is still a tremendous need for more and better programs and services.

Activists forging multidimensional collective action frames are often the "other" in multiple communities—lesbians among gay men, people of color among white gays, gay among straight people of color, and so on. Thus, the people they are attempting to "realign" are often both supportive and antagonistic. Partial oppositional consciousness necessitates collective action within marginalized communities, subsequently inhibiting to a significant degree direct protest against dominant institutions. However, expanding oppositional consciousness to be more encompassing strengthens the community's ability to launch more effective attacks against the power structure. Aldon Morris writes that "effective social protest informed by a mature oppositional consciousness enables challenging groups to strip away the garments of universality from hegemonic consciousness, revealing its essential characteristics" (Morris 1992: 370).

Of particular importance is the fact that such collective action is shaped by a strategy to build coalitions that rest upon the existing oppositional cultures of oppressed communities, thereby expanding this oppositional culture to include other forms of oppositional consciousness. In Chapter 3, activists of color employed elements of their oppositional racial cultures to promote pro-LGBT collective consciousness. In Chapter 4, prison AIDS activists linked symbols of queer resistance to raise consciousness about the oppression of prisoners with HIV/AIDS. These inclusive, multidimensional frame alignment processes draw on multiple cultures of resistance to simultaneously transform multiple oppressive beliefs, traditions, and practices.

5. *Multiple oppositional movements emerge in response to multiple inequalities, creating the possibility for positive cross-movement alliances.* Systems of oppression in the United States and other countries have been targeted by numerous oppositional movements. The 1960s and 1970s witnessed, among others, the women's movement, the movement against the Vietnam War, the Civil Rights movement, the black power movement, the Chicano/a movement, the gay liberation movement, and the American Indian Movement. In the 1990s, social movement activity included such issues as AIDS, LGBT rights, abortion rights, violence against women, police brutality, Puerto Rican independence, access for physically disabled people, environmental issues, and a revitalized interest in fighting globalization. Although multiple inequalities have promoted divisions between movements, they have also raised the potential for constructive alliances between movements.

My findings show that participants' prior political involvement in antiapartheid, antiracist, gay and lesbian, and feminist movements had a tremendous effect on AIDS activism. These activists served as *movement bridges,* using the ideological analyses and organizing skills learned in other movements to forge effective campaigns to fight AIDS. For example, Frank worked in several different movements, including the Civil Rights movement, the antiwar movement, the gay liberation movement, and the Puerto Rican independence movement. As an AIDS activist in the 1980s and the 1990s, he brought with him a sophisticated, radical political ideology and extensive organizing skills from other movements.

In contrast to those with no prior activist experience, AIDS movement participants with activist histories were more likely to make connections between the AIDS epidemic and systemic inequalities. Those activists immersed in other social movement communities were more likely to articulate multidimensional oppositional consciousness. The ideological tools they acquired in other movements facilitated their leadership in marginalized areas of the movement, such as HIV/AIDS among injection drug users, women, and prisoners.

In several cases, experienced activists chose to become involved in the AIDS movement because the AIDS crisis presented palpable manifestations of the intersections of multiple inequalities. In addition, participation in the AIDS movement led to a more inclusive oppositional consciousness for some participants. They were able to take their own experiences combating the AIDS crisis and apply them to other social problems. Today, many of them have continued to be active fighting AIDS as well as other social problems—utilizing the lessons they learned in the AIDS movement a decade ago. For example, five years after ACT UP/Chicago disbanded, I found one former member (and interview respondent) playing a leadership role in the wide array of progressive protests against the Democratic National Convention in Los Angeles in August 2000.

Of particular interest is the role that existing social movement networks and communities have played in the emergence of AIDS organizations. Feminist, antiracist, and gay and lesbian protest infrastructures were crucial in the formation of collective action targeting AIDS. As seen in Chapters 3 and 4, many AIDS activists have remained involved in various social movement communities. The networks, organizations, and participants in these communities have lent important resources to AIDS groups. Thus, social movement communities are clearly essential in sustaining collective action. Analyses that focus on particular social movements in isolation fail to capture the complex relationships among different oppositional movements.

Because it directly affects several marginalized communities, AIDS has provided the opportunity for relationships among different communities. Stoller writes: "Because it [AIDS] is a crisis that crosses divisions of race, gender, class, and sexuality, it can also bring people together across boundaries that usually separate movements for social change" (Stoller 1998: 154) Within ACT UP, there have been alliances between LGBTs and prisoners, recovering addicts, communities of color, and poor women (all of which are overlapping groups). In cities such as Los Angeles, different gay male communities of color found common cause in fighting AIDS, forming lasting coalitions and social networks. Thus, crosscutting issues such as AIDS create the possibility of alliances and coalitions—critically important social movement resources.

Future Research

By the year 2002, nearly 500,000 people had died of AIDS in the United States alone. Yet social movement scholars have paid minimal attention to the rich and varied aspects of the AIDS movement. One could argue that there is something to be learned about such a movement precisely because it so stigmatized. It is a movement that has wrestled with racism, sexism, homophobia, classism, addiction, incarceration, poverty, and globalization. The analysis here clearly demonstrates the critical importance of attention to multiple inequalities in the AIDS movement. Both the structural forces highlighted by resource mobilization theory and the social psychological forces emphasized by contemporary social movement theorists are mediated by multiple systems of oppression. These oppressions shape organizational development, access to resources, collective consciousness, strategies, tactics, and repression. In the year 2003, the infection of 30–40 million people in the third world begs a social movement analysis of international AIDS activism.

Hopefully, the future will see more social movement analyses of AIDS activism. Such studies will undoubtedly provide additional insight into the effect of multiple inequalities on collective action. The intersectional approach to collective action developed here is by no means only applicable to the AIDS movement. Sociological research focusing on both historical and contemporary movements will be enriched by attention to the interactions between multiple oppressions.

For example, as pointed out by Angela Davis (1983), the women's suffrage movement of the nineteenth century grew out of women's disaffection within the male-dominated abolitionist movement. An intersectional social movement approach could be used to investigate gender relations within the abolitionist movement and the events that led to the alienation of women in the movement. Such an approach could also shed light on the race and class dynamics within the suffrage movement that eventually led to its alliance with the racist eugenics movement in the early 1900s.

With some notable exceptions (e.g., Payne 1996) sociological research on the Civil Rights movement has often neglected the role that gender played throughout the movement. Looking at the Civil Rights movement in terms of only race or race and class provides only partial insight. Gender was an absolutely crucial factor in the development of the Civil Rights movement. As scholars outside sociology have shown, African American women formed the backbone of the movement, performing key organizing and protest tasks that often went unnamed (Giddings 1984; Davis 1983). In turn, sexism within organizations such as the Southern Christian Leadership Conference and the Student Nonviolent Coordinating Committee restricted the opportunities of women activists, thereby reducing the overall potential of the movement and simultaneously sowing the seeds for a new wave of feminism.

The emergence of black feminism in the 1970s was linked to sexism within the Civil Rights movement and the black power movement as well as racism and classism within the women's movement. Black lesbians also brought their experiences with homophobic oppression to the table (Smith 1983, 1993). Black feminists have been at the forefront in developing interactive analyses of power as well as forging interactive strategies for resistance. Research by social movement theorists on the development of black feminism—as theory and practice—would provide invaluable knowledge concerning the relationships among multiple inequalities and their impact on collective action.

An intersectional approach is especially powerful in studying social movement activity as we move forward in the twenty-first century. In addition to the AIDS movement, other contemporary movements are shaped by multiple inequalities. Battles for reproductive rights revolve not just around gender issues but also race and class. Poor women and women of color have been historically targeted with sterilization abuse and continue to be disproportionately affected by restricted access to abortion. Interestingly, "pro-life" leaders have often appropriated the language and tactics of the Civil Rights movement. They have also appealed to African Americans by equating abortion with racial genocide. These are just two of the ways in which this current issue is shaped by intersectionality.

The ideological and organizational overlap between the opponents of abortion rights and LGBT rights highlights the links between patriarchy and heterosexism. For example, the Catholic Church has been a pivotal force in opposing the AIDS movement, abortion rights, and LGBT rights. Social movement analyses would be advanced greatly by examining the role of the Catholic Church in sexist and homophobic countermovements. These are just a few of the forms of collective action that can be more fully understood from an intersectional theoretical perspective.

Lessons for Fighting HIV/AIDS

In addition to building upon social movement theory, the research and analysis presented here presents fundamental lessons for people organizing to combat the AIDS crisis and other social problems fueled by multiple oppressions. In terms of understanding the AIDS crisis, the data reaffirm several points stressed by many AIDS activists worldwide. One critical lesson is that a purely biological understanding of AIDS (or tuberculosis, or other contagious diseases) is inadequate in formulating ways to fight the disease. The spread of the virus has been catalyzed by systemic oppression for over two decades. If inequality—in all its forms, on both institutional and ideological levels—is not attacked, more and more people will get infected and die. This is particularly true in the year 2003, as new infections among poor African Americans and Latinos—particularly gay and bisexual men and injection drug users—have come to compose an even larger proportion of the total cases of HIV infection and AIDS. On the international level, many less industrialized countries, particularly in sub-Saharan Africa, are currently being decimated by AIDS—a decimation directly linked to an inequitable global, capitalist economy (Farmer 1996).

Challenging the social domination intertwined with the spread of AIDS necessitates grassroots action. The history of the crisis has demonstrated that waiting for those in power to develop effective AIDS programs and services is deadly: "Silence = Death."

Tremendous gains have come from confrontational protest that has forced institutions such as the government, the medical establishment, the media, and pharmaceutical corporations to expend greater resources to combat HIV/AIDS. Although it is important to be aware of the differential costs of participation, direct action, including civil disobedience, is still required to truly end the AIDS crisis.

ACT UP was undoubtedly the most important organization in waking up a country blinded to the needless loss of hundreds of thousands of lives. As we begin the twenty-first century, the ACT UP model of intensive research and documentation, bold statements of queer pride, and direct action continues to hold promise for change. There is still a need to force pharmaceutical companies and government researchers to look at alternative avenues for fighting HIV and to increase access to health care. The current legislative attempts to further curtail the rights of LGBT communities and communities of color, as well as budget cuts on welfare, health care, and other social programs, are particularly threatening in the face of continued high rates of HIV infection in diverse communities. AIDS activism must target all forms of oppression related to the epidemic.

These struggles must also occur within other AIDS organizations and affected communities. The internal divisions in ACT UP and other groups reflect the systems of oppression in larger society. Undoubtedly, the ideological and strategic framework of groups like ACT UP needs to be further expanded and modified to be more inclusive of race, class, gender, and related issues of power (e.g., immigrant status), all of which have been and continue to be critical factors in the epidemiology of AIDS. Likewise, organizations within and outside the LGBT community need to be more aggressive in creatively challenging homophobia and the broader antisex morality that continue to contribute to the spread of the HIV virus.

In addition to instrumental activism, there is a need for community-based organizations to be controlled by people directly affected by HIV/AIDS, including not only people living with HIV/AIDS but their family members, friends, and political comrades. Community-based efforts must be guided by dialogue, indigenous cultural traditions, empowerment, and inclusivity. These initiatives must take into account the impact of social location—what "isms" people deal with and what daily problems they face. They include not only concrete problems such as housing, addiction, immigrant status, employment, and health care but also internalized oppression. Indeed, individual and collective empowerment are indispensable components in confronting AIDS.

Awareness of social location means recognizing that people do not always fit neatly into one particular social group. Efforts to promote collective consciousness must take into account dual identities, such as being LGBT and of color. Various types of AIDS programs must be coordinated to adequately handle the complicated situations of marginalized populations. A person with HIV/AIDS may be both a former prisoner and an addict. Thus, HIV/AIDS agencies must be able to deal with issues facing prisoners, addicts, and people with chronic mental illness. Women at risk for HIV infection are sometimes both sex workers and mothers. They are sometimes lesbian injection drug users. Prevention and intervention efforts must deal with such multiple economic and social realities. In 2003, HIV/AIDS-related care frequently continues to be fragmented and ill-equipped to deal with multiply marginalized groups.

A key element in successful AIDS activism is building alliances between different sectors of the movement and with other movements. Coalitions are necessary to maximize resources, share information, and form a broad political base capable of disrupting business as usual and wresting concrete concessions from the powers that be. They are also necessary to resist attempts by authorities to repress such activism. Because the HIV virus has directly affected so many different communities, the potential for coalition building is particularly powerful. For example, alliances with people fighting for a national health care plan and reproductive rights for women, as well as against the prison industrial complex, should be used to strengthen organized opposition to oppression.

Though the road ahead is still rocky, to say the least, AIDS activist campaigns have yielded many positive outcomes. Individuals at risk for HIV infection have been empowered, as seen in widespread safer sex practices and higher rates of HIV testing. People living with HIV/AIDS in the United States now have greater access to a larger number of treatments. Many people living with HIV/AIDS have become active participants in their own treatment and are living longer and more productive lives. Many people affected by HIV/AIDS have challenged internalized oppression, and many have become involved as peer educators, counselors, advocates, and street-level activists. Direct action has forced dominant institutions to expend more resources on HIV/AIDS. HIV/AIDS-related discrimination and prejudice have been significantly reduced. These are just a few of the ways in which the AIDS movement has been successful.

The battles being fought on racial, gender, and sexual fronts give us a good look at how AIDS activists have attempted to transform the collective consciousness of different sectors of society. In addition to creating mechanisms for prevention and AIDS care, AIDS activism has continued to chip away at racism, homophobia, sexism, and classism in different marginalized communities themselves. Within communities of color, inroads have been made in challenging sexism and homophobia as well as bridging class divisions. Within the LGBT community, AIDS activists have made progress in battling racism, sexism, and classism. All in all, these changes are crucial in developing a united front capable of bringing about a more fundamental transformation of society.

The organizations studied here have developed an extensive set of tactics that pay attention to the social aspects of AIDS. In turn, these tactics may be instructive for people working on other social problems that may also be the product of multiple forms of inequality (such as homelessness, substance abuse, incarceration, domestic violence, environmental injustice). In order to launch effective political struggles, agents for change must take into account these multiple oppressions and how they operate on micro- and macrolevels. Successful campaigns for change must assess which aspects of traditional culture reinforce current inequities and which can be tapped into to promote progressive change.

Politically, the AIDS movement demonstrated that singular approaches to oppression—be they narrowly LGBT, feminist, or antiracist—are likely to fail. In the face of interlocking inequalities, collective action that prioritizes one inequality as primary and others as inconsequential is more easily countered by elites. Such oppositional movements actually contribute to other forms of oppression by alienating valuable segments of marginalized communities. The oft-heard argument that we must tackle one particular form of domination "first" fails to acknowledge that different forms of domination are mutually reinforcing and often occur simultaneously. Only militant, united front strategies that take aim at all forms of oppression hold the promise of carving out a more just and humane society.

However, some will likely argue that a multidimensional oppositional consciousness will dilute the effectiveness of collective action. For example, an organization might attempt to initiate so many campaigns targeting various issues that it fails to be successful in any of them. However, I think this is more an issue of overextending the group's resources than of consciousness. Multidimensional oppositional consciousness, as I have defined it, does not require one organization to take on all the problems of the world but to be aware of the many ways in which oppressions interact. Key to such a consciousness is inclusion. A group might focus on only one issue but be very inclusive with respect to that issue. For example, a group of feminists might choose to organize around domestic violence. Here, "inclusion" means being cognizant of the challenges facing not only middle-class heterosexual women who speak English, but poor women, immigrant women, lesbians, monolingual Spanish speakers, and so on.

Such inclusion is key in all areas of progressive and radical organizing. As LGBT movements gain ground around the world, it has become even more important to recognize that most queers are not white or affluent. The "lesbian and gay rights movement" has of late developed campaigns that have paid little attention to issues of race, class, and globalization. For example, the campaign to end discrimination against lesbians and gay men in the U.S. military has consistently failed to critique the military as an oppressive force used by the U.S. government and multinational corporations to maintain U.S. economic interests in the Middle East, Latin America, Asia, and other places. This military force has led to the deaths of millions—both queer and straight—around the world, most recently thousands of Afghan civilians.

The ongoing campaign for "gay and lesbian marriage" ignores the fact that having the right to get married will not help poor queers to rise out of poverty or significantly increase their access to quality health care. A more inclusive strategy might perhaps be to strive for a national health care plan so that people in the United States would have access to health care, whether they were married or not.

Taking part in some of the antiglobalization mass marches that have occurred since 1999, I have been excited to see queer contingents loudly condemning U.S. policies that impoverish and brutalize people around the world. I have also been pleasantly surprised to see *some* straight activists recognize the need to fight homophobia—in their own communities and around the world—as part of any international movement for justice and peace. However, far too few mainstream LGBT activists see the links between homophobia and other oppressions, and far too many ostensibly progressive and radical straight activists (be they people of color or white; poor, working-class, or affluent) ignore homophobia as a system of oppression. Both of these tendencies only serve to promote disunity and inhibit coalition building. It remains to be seen how the numerous movements in the United States and around the world will interact in the years to come. On this subject, George Carter writes that direct action "requires coalition-building and communication with other people, persuasions, cultures—it requires solidarity. It is clear that we live in a world of interlocking systems; it is no longer possible to view the world solely on the basis of isolated problems" (Carter 1992: 21).

This recognition of "a world of interlocking systems" is critical for those U.S. activists working in solidarity with AIDS activists in other countries, particularly developing nations. More than 95 percent of all HIV-infected people now live in "developing" nations, which have also experienced 95 percent (over 20 million) of all AIDS deaths (Centers for Disease Control 2001). Globally, AIDS activists are currently going up against the enormous political and economic power of pharmaceutical companies (and the global "free trade" entities that assist them) that are working to prevent the production of generic antivirals for people with HIV/AIDS in poor nations. In addition, these AIDS activists must contend with histories of colonialism as well as current neocolonial economic policies (e.g., structural adjustment policies that prohibit governments from investing in national health care) that fuel the AIDS crisis, particularly in sub-Saharan Africa (see Schoepf, Schoepf, and Millen 2000). Thus, global AIDS activists and antiglobalization activists have much in common and stand to gain by expanding their coalitions.

* * *

Whether analyzing the birth of new movements, collective consciousness, strategies and tactics, internal conflict, coalitions, or repression, an intersectional approach is essential for critical social movement scholarship. Interlocking oppressions interact on societal, community, and movement levels to impede collective action. These multiple oppressions make social movements vulnerable to internal conflict as well as external repression. In response, remarkable activists like Catalina, Jeff, Frank, Phil, Javier, and others engage in community- and movement-level activism to promote a more inclusive oppositional consciousness while simultaneously challenging multiple oppressions on the institutional level. In addition to tackling the immediate crisis of HIV and AIDS, these and other activists welded together different oppositional consciousnesses, united cultures of resistance, and carved out protest infrastructures that were and continue to be capable of attacking multiple forms of oppression that are at the core of the AIDS crisis and numerous other social and public health problems.

Appendix A:
List of Organizations

ACT UP (AIDS Coalition to Unleash Power), Los Angeles, New York City, Chicago
AIDS Counseling and Education (ACE), Bedford Hills, New York
AIDS Foundation of Chicago
AIDS in Prison Project, New York City
AIDS Legal Council, Chicago
AIDS Project Los Angeles
American Indian House, New York City
Asian Pacific Islander Coalition on HIV/AIDS, New York City
Black AIDS Mobilization (BAM!), New York City
Caribbean Women's Health Association, Brooklyn
Chicago Women's AIDS Project
Gay and Lesbian Latino AIDS Education Initiative, Philadelphia
Gay Men of Color Consortium, Los Angeles:
- AIDS Prevention Team
- Asian Pacific AIDS Intervention Team
- Bienestar
- Minority AIDS Project
- Teatro Viva
Gay Men's Health Crisis, New York City
Kupona Network, Chicago
Prisoners with AIDS Rights Advocacy Group (PWA RAG), Atlanta

Recovery Alliance, Chicago
Shanti Project, Los Angeles
Southeast Michigan AIDS Alliance, Detroit
Stop AIDS, Chicago
VIDA/SIDA (Puerto Rican AIDS project), Chicago
Women in the Director's Chair, Chicago
Women's Health Education Project, Chicago

Appendix B:
Interview Questions

1. Demographics: Respondent's self-reported race and ethnicity, sex, sexuality, class, and current organizational affiliation.
2. What social change organizations have you been involved in (other than AIDS)? Describe your experiences.
   - What made you get involved?
   - Group composition (race, class, gender, sexuality)
   - Type (grassroots, private, nonprofit, etc.)
   - Philosophy, goals
   - Issues: Did the group do any AIDS work?
   - Strategies, tactics
   - Was the group successful in achieving established goals?
   - Problems you encountered
   - Have your organizational experiences affected the way you think and how you live your life?
3. What made you get involved in AIDS activism?
4. Describe the AIDS organizations you have been in or are involved with now.
   - How did you get involved?
   - How did the organization get started? Who started it? Did other organizations play a role in its formation?
   - Structure: membership, leadership (hierarchical vs. decentralized)
   - Philosophy, goals

- Issues: Which issues are priorities?
- How are decisions made?
- Strategies: What are the group's long-term strategies? Where do you focus your energy?
- Resources (financial and other), sources
- How do you get people involved?
- Tactics: What kind?

5. What external factors have made fighting AIDS more or less difficult?
   - Aspects of the different communities that help or hinder organizing
   - Gay communities of color, white gay and lesbian communities, heterosexual communities of color, other communities
   - Relationships with other groups, alliances—supportive, antagonistic?
   - How have government policies affected the group? Do you see any change with the Clinton presidential administration?
   - Successes or failures of group?
   - Repression, pressure to tone down?
   - Do you have any criticisms of the group?

6. What are some of the things you think are important for the AIDS movement?
   - Ideology
   - Organizational composition: What kind of organizations are the most useful?
   - Alliances, coalition work
   - Strategies; any links to other issues or movements; dealing with racism, sexism, homophobia
   - Tactics

7. What do you think has been the role of direct action in the AIDS movement?
   - How would you describe the relationship between direct action groups like ACT UP and other segments of the AIDS movement—in particular, grassroots service groups and large AIDS agencies? Do you think this situation should change?
   - What do you see as the "ACT UP" model? Can this approach be utilized in communities outside the white gay male community? Explain.
   - Have you been to a demonstration or other direct action event? As part of an organization or as an individual?
   - How does having a job in the AIDS arena affect direct action activism?

8. Miscellaneous:
   - Is there anything you'd like to add? Questions or perspectives that are missing from the interview? Suggestions for my research?
   - Do you know anyone you think I should interview? Organizations I should contact?

Appendix C:
ACT UP/Chicago's
World AIDS Day Leaflet

Illinois Prisoner Statements
World AIDS Day, December 1, 1994

ACT UP/Chicago has been working with Illinois prisoners to fight HIV and AIDS in Illinois prisons. A prisoner-conducted study at one correctional facility found that 65% of inmates surveyed received no counseling before or after their HIV antibody test. 76% would like to learn more about AIDS. 63% think condoms should be allowed in prison. 87% believe prisoners should be allowed to participate in new clinical trials and treatment. Through letters and phone calls, prisoners have documented current conditions and have been instrumental in formulating demands to improve AIDS programs. Below are excerpts from letters received from prisoners.

Since I been incarcerated it seems like everyone I know just abandoned me. No one comes to visit me or even send me a letter. . . . Some people think that if they touch me that they will become infected with the HIV.

The majority of those inmates are not using any kind of protection. . . . And if something isn't done real soon the situation is going to get totally out of control. And that is why prisoners desperately need prevention and awareness programs. And don't you think for one minute that it is just ignorance and lack of money on the part of the prison administration that such programs are not already implemented. Instead, the bottom line here in prison is—they do not care. If five hundred inmates were to die tomorrow, the cells would be refilled before the week was out. . . . Believe me, these people are not in any hurry to combat HIV and the spread of AIDS.

At this present time, the only information the prisoners here get on the deadly disease is from the television. Other than that, there really isn't much more information available. It is really a shame that we don't have some kind of AIDS awareness program here.

I asked the warden to put condoms in the commissary, but they refused because they say it would only promote more sex between inmates. That's a joke, believe me. These people condone unsafe sex every day on visits and at picnics.

My pretest counseling consisted of being told to sign a sheet of paper so I could be tested. When I asked why I was being tested, the response was that it was requested. I still haven't found out who requested the test. The post-test counseling consisted of being shown a piece of paper which said "non-reactive," whatever that means.

On February 3, 1992, I was advised by the doctor here that I was HIV-positive. Since I was being released the next day, I was, naturally, devastated. In reviewing the medical records, there is every indication that the medical staff was aware as early as May of 1991. Having experienced several medical problems, my T-cell count was 418 on May 5, 1991; 311 on December 16, 1991; and 427 on January 2, 1992. During this, I was not made aware of my HIV problem and wasn't given any medication.

I was diagnosed as being HIV-positive in 1991. I have been incarcerated since 1992. This is the most corrupt and inefficient ran prison in the state. Ex: My condition requires that I have blood work drawn every three months to monitor my T-cell count, etc. I'm also suppose to be seen by the doctor to discuss my lab results and given a routine checkup. None of the above has been done in four and a half months now. . . . When I run out of medication it takes them two weeks to issue me more.

The medical staff discuss my medical information with non-medical staff. I'm discriminated against about where I'm to be placed on visit. Almost everyone in the joint know about my illness. I didn't tell them—the medical staff did.

After having gone over World Health Organization guidelines on HIV infection and AIDS in prisons, I've noticed that not only has IDOC ignored their suggestions of condom distribution and peer educators, but also: support when prisoners are notified of test results and in the period following; effective viricidal agent, with instructions on cleaning injecting equipment; access to information on treatment options, and access to clinical trials of treatments for all HIV/AIDS-related diseases. . . . Unless the Illinois Department of Corrections seriously addresses condom distribution and a comprehensive education and prevention program, the HIV/AIDS epidemic in prisons will become far worse and more costly later on.

I have HIV. . . . There's no one in prison who speaks or shows concern for people with AIDS. There's no hope or help for our families. There's no dietary program for people with AIDS. I'm supposed to avoid stress. I'm so far from home that I and my family worry all the time. There's no one here that I can voice my concerns to. I'm always told that "we're working on it."

* * *

The Dying Room

They say that a man's not supposed to cry
Especially not men like ourselves.
Locked down in prison, away from the world
In our own very private
And incomplete hells.

There's a place here I know, that no one wants to go
And I'll tell you the sad reason why,
This is a place, where the body goes to waste
It's a room in the hospital
Where they put you to die.

The place where I reside is a place for those souls
Who are sentenced, and must serve out their time,
We are convicts all . . . and that's true enough
Yet sometimes, another's sadness,
Gets mixed up with mine.

Even the coldest hearts ache, for a poor soul's sake
Who has only a short time to live.
It's a shame when your demise is institutionalized
So the state can get all
That your soul has to give.

This puts me in mind
Of the dark, grim reaper
Pulling the skin from the bones
Of the non-believer.

This practice is real, it's alive and well
And it's time that we asked ourselves why,
Why does one's days, have to just sliver away
In that blue room where they put you
When it is time for you to die. . . .

—written by a prisoner in an Illinois state prison

Notes

Chapter 1

1. The publishing records of *ASR, JAS,* and *Social Forces* are only slightly worse than other journals, such as *Sociological Quarterly* and *Sociological Perspectives,* which published, respectively, three articles and one article on HIV/AIDS between 1986 and 1999. The *Journal of Health and Social Behavior,* which one would think would be a logical place for articles focusing on an epidemic that has killed tens of millions worldwide, published a mere sixteen articles during the same fourteen-year period (Lichenstein 2001).

2. Nancy Stoller's 1998 book, *Lessons from the Damned,* provides an intersectional (attentive to multiple, intersecting systems of inequality) analysis of several distinct AIDS organizing initiatives.

3. Here it is important to note that, in my book, I speak of the AIDS movement in the past tense because, although extremely valuable AIDS activism still occurs, there is no longer a national, mass-based grassroots movement. For example, ACT UP, the largest grassroots organization in the AIDS movement, was largely defunct by 1995 (Cohen 1998; Gould 2000). Other smaller organizations that engaged in social protest, such as Black AIDS Mobilization (BAM!), or advocated more radical political perspectives, such as Prisoners with AIDS Rights Advocacy Group (PWA RAG) have disappeared. In turn, as Patton (1990) noted over a decade ago, many grassroots AIDS service organizations became increasingly institutionalized during the 1980s. The 1990s witnessed further bureaucratization and a parallel shift away from protest within many AIDS agencies.

4. I am not arguing that these other inequalities played no role in the earliest years; they did. However, historically, homophobia was the central

oppressive system that patterned initial responses to the AIDS crisis in the United States.

5. Some "men who have sex with men" (MSM) do not identify as gay or bisexual. However, my own experience "identifying" as heterosexual and then bisexual, followed by seventeen years living as an "out" gay man and living and working in several gay communities, leads me to believe that a rather large proportion of these men would like to be able to identify as gay men if homophobia were not so pervasive. The origins of the term "men who have sex with men" are insightful here. Black gay activist Phil Wilson, speaking with Cathy Cohen about (Cohen's words) "controversial compromises of black gay activists" to acquire CDC funding, stated:

> The other thing we did out of our naivete, is that we came up with this phrase, "men who have sex with men." Quite frankly it was a phrase that was created by black gay men, and we created it because we knew that the CDC would not fund black gay men. So we wanted to create a phrase that was palatable to them. In the beginning we created it out of the air. There was no statistical work done to quantify the magnitude of this population of black men who were having sex with other men but didn't identify. Now intuitively we knew that they were engaged in homosexual behavior. However, the way that behavior manifested itself was not, or did not mirror the way it manifested itself in white gay men. But now the implication that there are no black gay men out there who identify as gay is absurd. . . . Besides who are these men who have sex with men fucking anyway? They are fucking men who identify with being gay, that's who they are fucking. (Cohen 1999: 107–108)

My point here is that although "MSM" is sometimes a useful category, it often obscures and minimizes the existence of gay-identified men, particularly gay men of color.

6. Here, it is important to point out that Shilts's work itself often plays into the hands of homophobes by setting up dangerous categories of "good gays" and "bad gays." The "good gays" promote a "homosexual lifestyle" that mimics dominant heterosexual ideals, striving to assimilate into mainstream society. The "bad gays" (those termed "fast lane" gays by Shilts) engage in casual sex, their attitudes and behaviors challenging the rigid heterosexual ideology of monogamy.

7. Many gay men living with HIV/AIDS remain closeted about their status today, and challenging institutionalized bigotry and homophobic collective beliefs continues to be a necessary component of AIDS activism in 2003.

8. In this book, I sometimes use the term *queer* to refer to lesbian, gay, bisexual, and transgender individuals and organizations. The term is controversial within LGBT communities, with some folks seeing it as an affirming, inclusive, and defiant term and others seeing it as detracting from LGBT efforts to assimilate into mainstream heterosexual society.

9. A die-in occurs when protesters drop to the street (or office floor, etc.) during a march or a demonstration and lie down for a specified time period to dramatize lives lost to AIDS. A phone zap involves activists calling the

offices of a particular target repeatedly, often all day, in order to tie up the phone lines and disrupt "business as usual." Likewise, a fax zap overloads a target's fax machine.

10. Here, it is important to note that these different communities overlap; for example, there were gay male prisoners and former prisoners active in the Prisoner's with AIDS Rights Advocacy Group.

11. Regretfully, I was only able to interview two Native American AIDS activists for my study and thus my analysis focuses more on African Americans, Latinos/as, Asian Americans and Pacific Islanders, and whites.

12. This translates to a prevalence of AIDS that is at least fifteen times their proportion of the overall U.S. population.

13. This calculation assumes that about 10 percent of men in general are gay. The lower we make this "gay percentage" (or the percentage of MSM who are gay-identified), the more startling the proportion of African American gay men among the total number of people living with AIDS.

14. When I use the term *social movement theory,* I refer to the body of literature on social movements and collective action developed primarily by sociologists (and a few political scientists)—the vast majority of which is not read by social movement participants themselves. There is a wealth of substantive and theoretical work that has been written by activists and revolutionaries themselves (e.g., Malcolm X, Gloria Anzaldúa, Audre Lorde, Adrienne Rich, Frantz Fanon, Ernesto "Che" Guevara, Cindy Patton, Douglas Crimp, Angela Davis) that I consider to be very useful as an activist myself. In this book, I have attempted to bridge the gap between "activist" theory and "sociological" theory.

15. Political process frameworks challenge strands of resource mobilization theory that argue that third parties control social movements, arguing instead that movements are built primarily using *indigenous* resources. Research by Morris (1984) and McAdam (1982) reveals that organizational funding, group leaders, and members often come from within indigenous communities and that aspects of indigenous culture promote collective resistance. This research also indicates that social movement groups operate within a structure of political opportunities, attempting to exploit shifts in the political climate, demographic changes, and elite conflicts to promote social change.

16. In contrast to prior social psychological approaches, contemporary models centered on "frame alignment" (aligning potential participants' understandings of a particular social problem and related beliefs with those of the social movement organization) and "micromobilization" (how social movement organizations go about drawing people into collective action) attempt to link social psychological and structural processes (see essays in Morris and Mueller 1992).

17. There has been a good deal of research demonstrating the importance of oppositional culture and consciousness in modern social movements, including the Civil Rights movement (Carson 1996; Morris 1984; McAdam 1988), the black power movement (Allen 1992), the feminist movement (Echols 1989; Taylor 1989; Lengermann and Wallace 1985), the LGBT movement (Cruickshank 1992; Adam 1987; D'Emilio 1983; Deitcher 1995), and the labor movement (Fantasia 1989; Piven and Cloward 1977).

18. William Gamson suggests that changes at the cultural level be given the same status as institutional changes, stating that the "construction of a

collective identity is one step in challenging cultural domination" (W. Gamson 1992: 60).

19. When we look at AIDS activism through the lens of social movement theory, it is clear that the AIDS movement grew out of preexisting organizations and networks—consistent with resource mobilization models. Likewise, tactics and strategies have been central to movement outcomes. Consistent with contemporary social movement theory (W. Gamson 1992; Taylor and Whittier 1992; Klandermans 1992), collective action has targeted intertwined structural and ideological barriers. Research on AIDS activism by Josh Gamson (1989) and Stoller (1998) demonstrates the centrality of collective action frames (ways in which groups of people perceive social problems and possible strategies for change) as conceptualized by Tarrow (1992). Scholarship on the AIDS movement (Corea 1992; Arno and Feiden 1992; essays in ACT UP/New York 1992) indicates that collective action has occurred within networks equivalent to the social movement communities described by Taylor and Whittier (1992). These social movement communities engage in frame alignment processes, in particular frame transformation (Snow et al. 1986). Within the AIDS movement, there is clear evidence that battles over social meaning (e.g., debates over clean needle exchanges) have been at the center ring and that cultural change (e.g., promoting more positive perceptions of homosexuality) has been inextricably linked to institutional change (Klandermans 1992; W. Gamson 1992).

20. Thus, "frame alignment" (Snow et al. 1986) and other approaches (McAdam 1982; W. Gamson 1989; Klandermans 1988; Melucci 1989) that attempt to explain how social movement organizations challenge dominant ideology and mobilize new movement participants do not account for the impact of multiple forms of oppression and consciousness.

21. The theoretical concept of multiple interlocking systems of oppression has been introduced into the field of sociology by black feminist sociologists such as Deborah King (1988) and Patricia Hill Collins (1990). While interactive theoretical frameworks such as "black feminism," "multiracial feminism," and "intersectionality" have often been marginalized within the discipline of sociology, the 1990s witnessed an increase in scholarship in these areas (e.g., Collins 1993; Zinn and Dill 1997; Lorber 2001).

22. For example, Barbara Smith (1983) notes that black feminists have been involved in a variety of social change efforts, including reproductive rights, health care, child care, the rights of the disabled, violence against women, welfare rights, lesbian and gay rights, educational reform, housing, women in prison, aging, police brutality, labor organizing, anti-imperialist struggles, antiracist organizing, nuclear disarmament, and environmental justice.

23. I would argue that by the late 1990s, there was no "AIDS movement" in the United States. AIDS-related services became increasingly bureaucratized and less community-based as the AIDS crisis continued. By the mid-1990s, most ACT UP chapters and other direct action groups had ceased to exist. Today, many activists derisively refer to the "AIDS industry" and decry the lack of grassroots activism because certain communities are still underserved and people are still dying of AIDS. However, AIDS *activism* continues to be a potent social force.

24. An additional interview was conducted in Detroit, Michigan. Another was conducted by phone with a prisoner in an Illinois state prison.

Chapter 2

1. On the other hand, many ACT UP activists had never participated in activism before ACT UP. See Elbaz (1992) and Cohen (1998).

2. The close links between the LGBT community and AIDS activism is highlighted quite well by the thoughts of one of the few heterosexuals interviewed. Kate remarked: "Many people don't believe I'm straight and don't understand why I want to do this work." This included some ACT UP members, some of whom, according to Kate, thought she was closeted. She stated: "If I had any insecurities or any homophobia, I would have left. . . . If I was insecure with who I was, it would be really hard for me to do this work as a straight person."

3. Thus, radicals in ACT UP, for example, might disagree with Maria's suggestion to focus on heart disease.

4. This included extremely valuable work done by gay men of color, work that has often been overlooked by both white gay activists and AIDS scholars.

5. Although interracial relationships do not inherently have such power imbalances, many gay male activists of color with whom I have spoken observe that in many of these relationships, the white partner dominates the relationship economically and socially and that both partners negate the importance of the man of color's racial heritage and his experiences with racism. Of course, all relationships are unique—whether interracial or not. It would be interesting to interview gay men in interracial (or cross-class) relationships (involving the full spectrum of races) to analyze their experiences, motivations, and attitudes about their relationships.

6. Ken, a black gay man, reported that the Majority Action Committee (composed primarily of people of color) of ACT UP/New York asked for $11,000 to develop posters, advertisements for black and Latino/a publications, and other outreach materials to publicize upcoming planning meetings, educational forums, and demonstrations focusing on AIDS among people of color, especially women. Though ACT UP/New York had quickly passed a proposal for a $25,000 ad in the *New York Times* a month before, there was "much resistance" from the general body, and according to Ken, it took three weeks of coming back to the general body meetings and arguing with "ignorant" and "disrespectful" white members before the organization narrowly voted for the funds.

7. See Cohen (1999) for an examination of this dynamic in the black community of New York City.

8. Cohen notes that sexuality issues in general have played a role in African American communities' responses to the AIDS crisis:

We must remember that sexuality, or what has been defined by the dominant society as the abnormal sexuality of both black men and women (e.g., images such as oversexed black men in search of white women, promiscuous black women, and illegitimate baby producers), has been used to justify the implementation of marginalizing systems ranging from slavery to, most recently, workfare. . . . With such a history of marginalization in mind, we can begin to understand, yet never condone, how homophobia along with other systems of exclusion might be willingly deployed by black elites in an attempt to distance "the community" from blame and stigma and to retain their hopes of legitimacy and full incorporation. (Cohen 1999: 35)

9. One possible explanation for this disparity is that middle-class whites may have much less substantial contact with working-class and poor whites than middle-class people of color have with working-class and poor people of color. As Collins (1990) notes, many middle-class African Americans have extended family members who are working class or poor.

10. This reflects a dynamic common among progressive and radical organizers (both people of color and middle- and upper-class whites), particularly in urban areas: the failure to be cognizant of the economic marginalization of millions of poor and working-class whites.

11. This dichotomous thinking surfaced in earlier movements as well. Frank, who worked with the Black Panther Party in the early 1970s, noted that the Panthers respected and supported the gay liberation movement only to the extent that it was white and that the Panthers tended to deny the existence of black gay men and lesbians.

12. From a slightly different angle, one could argue that such an "antiracist" consciousness is not truly "antiracist" (nor fully oppositional) if it does not promote the autonomy and liberation of all people of color—including LGBT people of color.

13. Noel's resentment of "the self-appointed white lesbian and gay leaders" and his ideological connection to black political struggles also further complicate the issue of using African American movements (or other prominent movements) as reference points to legitimize another struggle. What might be the reactions of African American activists to parallels made between African American and Asian American social movements? What seems to be obscured at times is the fact that there are historical connections between the Civil Rights movement and gay and lesbian political struggles. The Civil Rights movement provided strategic and ideological models for other movements (McAdam 1988), including gay and lesbian rights movements. Many activists—black and white—who went on to fight for gay liberation received training in the trenches of the southern Civil Rights movement (D'Emilio 1983). Furthermore, many white lesbian and gay activists, as well as many African American heterosexual activists, often fail to recognize the remarkable efforts of lesbian and gay African Americans, such as James Baldwin, Audre Lorde, Bayard Rustin, and Barbara Smith, who have worked to bridge the gap between antiracist and antihomophobic struggles.

14. The concept of partial oppositional consciousness challenges the rigid dichotomization of the cultural-personal level and institutional level found in much social movement literature by illuminating the links between

social structure, collective identity, and individual biographies. More specifically, partial oppositional consciousness goes beyond Antonio Gramsci's (1987) hegemonic ideology and similar concepts by allowing for multiple, interactive forms of consciousness.

15. This reinforces the contention that both social problems (Spector and Kitsuse 1987) and social movements (Klandermans 1992) are socially constructed. The social categories upon which inequitable social systems are based are not natural but are produced by particular historical and structural conditions. Thus, these categories can be challenged and transformed, and corresponding identities will evolve.

Chapter 3

1. Dental dams are square pieces of latex traditionally used by dentists during dental procedures that can also be used to prevent HIV transmission during oral-anal and oral-vaginal sex.

2. Resource mobilization theories stress the centrality of strategies and tactics (Morris and Herring 1987; McAdam, McCarthy, and Zald 1988). Sociological research providing support for resource mobilization theories has focused on collective action utilizing "instrumental" tactics that are designed to effect change on an institutional level (e.g., sit-ins to integrate public accommodations, picketing to oppose discriminatory practices). "New" social movement theory and related social psychological approaches assert the importance of "prefigurative politics" or "identity politics" that stress the importance of cultural change (e.g., consciousness-raising groups to help women recognize their collectively experienced inequality) (Habermas 1981; Cohen 1985; Taylor and Whittier 1992; W. Gamson 1992).

3. The need to promote a sense of entitlement among people with HIV and AIDS challenges resource mobilization theories that typically treat grievances and discontent as given rather than as shaped by collective and individual meanings, ideas, and values (Mueller 1992). In addition, efforts to facilitate empowerment also demonstrate that forging oppositional consciousness involves not only culture but the social position (with respect to multiple oppressions) of potential movement participants. Frame alignment analyses (Snow et al. 1986) should therefore be expanded to grapple with the concrete conditions resulting from these multiple inequalities.

4. One gay Latino activist asserted: "The exclusion of gay men of color in mainstream ads in gay magazines is not seen by most white men as racist, but merely circumstantial."

5. It is important to note that there were people of color in ACT UP who were firmly rooted in various communities of color. Sometimes white ACT UP members' lack of support for this racial commitment led to racial conflict, as was the case in New York City, where black members left ACT UP to form BAM!

6. The efforts of lesbians and gay men of color to achieve community embeddedness shed light on the relationship between fostering multidimensional oppositional consciousness and movement concepts such as "multiorganizational fields" (Klandermans 1992) and "communities of challengers"

(Lo 1992). For a discussion of these concepts within the context of this data and in particular a critique of Lo's conceptualizations of "community" and "challengers," see Stockdill (2001a).

7. One important factor that Snow and Benford link to social movement success is "narrative fidelity," which they define as "the degree to which proffered framings resonate with cultural narrations . . . that are part and parcel of one's cultural heritage and thus function to inform events and experiences in the immediate present" (Snow and Benford 1988: 210).

8. As Cohen (1999) points out, class oppression exists *within* black communities. Classism is less likely to operate on the interpersonal and family level than homophobia and sexism but rather creates rifts between class-based African American communities.

9. This process can be seen as a synthesis of "frame bridging" and "frame transformation" (Snow and Benford 1988).

10. This is not to say that middle-class, white, ACT UP members did not have similar problems. They too had to do a great deal of organizing and mobilizing work to get their brothers and sisters to move beyond service provision and into the street. However, the intersection of multiple oppressions made community-level efforts even more complex for LGBTs of color.

11. Respondents reported two additional factors related to the lack of direct action regarding AIDS: the fact that AIDS is only one of numerous social problems devastating communities of color (see Chapter 2 and Chapter 5) and the increased likelihood of police brutality and imprisonment of activists of color (see Chapter 5).

Chapter 4

1. This is not to say that prisoners have not organized against oppression. Solidarity work from the outside would be impossible without the activism of prisoners behind the walls. For example, see ACT UP/New York (1992) for a description of AIDS organizing by women prisoners.

2. Statistics for Asian Americans, Pacific Islanders, and Native Americans were not provided by this source.

3. Conversation with activist and former prisoner Linda Evans (November 16, 2001). A 1998 report written by William Burdon and myself, entitled "HIV-related Programs and Policies of the Los Angeles County Jail System and the Conditions Facing Inmates Living with HIV/AIDS" (prepared for the HIV/AIDS Services for the Incarcerated Evaluation Committee, Los Angeles County Commission on HIV Health Services), documents systemic inadequacies in AIDS health care and AIDS-related services in the Los Angeles County Jail.

4. As seen in Chapter 3, race is also an important factor, with many gay men of color displaying multidimensional oppositional consciousness.

5. In this way, it was distinct not only from elite groups but from the movement halfway houses described by Morris. He defines a movement halfway house as "an established group or organization that is only partially integrated into the larger society because its participants are actively involved in efforts to bring about a desired change in society" (Morris 1984:

139). Although the Prison Issues Committee was not a movement halfway house, Morris's distinction between resources provided by those who identify with the goals of the movement and other political actors is a valuable one that presents a more complex picture of different social movement actors and organizations.

6. The term *dyke,* historically a derogatory reference to lesbians, has been reclaimed and used by many lesbians as a symbol of defiance and pride.

7. This supports the work of Taylor and Whittier who argue that "lesbian feminist communities sustain a collective identity that encourages women to engage in a wide range of social and political actions that challenge the dominant system" (Taylor and Whittier 1992: 105).

Chapter 5

1. Piven and Cloward's (1977) book, *Poor People's Movements,* suggests that state suppression is used in concert with other elite responses such as cooptation to undermine oppositional movements that threaten the status quo.

2. In some cases, the costs of participation are perceived to be so low that repression is not a factor in the decision to participate. For example, repression was found to be insignificant in decisions to sign a petition in support of the Dutch peace movement (Oegema and Klandermans 1994) and participating in the East German "revolution" of 1989 (Opp and Gern 1993).

3. Although repression may work in the interests of elites under some conditions, it may backfire in others and actually benefit social movements. Rick Fantasia's (1989) study of U.S. labor movements shows that arrests and police harassment may intimidate potential participants but at other times may galvanize worker solidarity. Brutality and violence on the part of authorities may lead previously neutral parties to support the movement (McAdam 1982; McAdam, McCarthy, and Zald 1988). In such cases, images of repression by the state—often filtered through the media—promote sympathy among the general public and important social groups. There is little evidence of this dynamic in the data for my study, which makes sense because I studied activists, not the general public. Although my data do not provide insight into why repression against ACT UP did not generate support outside the group, I would speculate that the following interrelated factors merit examination: (1) the general conservative political climate during the Reagan and George H. W. Bush administrations, (2) minimal and distorted corporate media coverage of ACT UP's activism, (3) homophobia and ignorance about HIV/AIDS that promoted fear and blame rather than compassion for people with HIV/AIDS, and (4) ACT UP's (and other groups') relative success in educating the public about AIDS and forcing the government to increase funding for AIDS. This last factor might very well have led many to think that there was little need for protest because the epidemic was "under control"

4. I would like to thank radical activist and scholar Debbie Gould for making this important observation during a conversation this past year.

5. More research is needed to contrast the reluctance of many African Americans and others to engage in civil disobedience and get arrested today,

versus the willingness of thousands of blacks to be arrested (and many severely beaten) during the Civil Rights movement. Although knowledge of increasing government violence during the 1960s is one factor, other factors might include changes in policing practices, the class makeup of those arrested, and media coverage.

6. Plastic handcuffs can indeed hurt, but they reflect the routinization of civil disobedience in which the police (and the government) see less of a threat from protestors.

7. It is significant that many of the most strident advocates of direct action in the study were Puerto Rican independence activists, a fact that reflects the ongoing militant struggle for Puerto Rican independence, particularly in New York and Chicago.

8. Maria, a Puerto Rican activist in New York City who had been arrested at a protest before, stated that if she were to get arrested again, it would be for an action connected to a larger political strategy, specifically the Puerto Rican independence movement.

9. Criminal prosecution in this case is not limited to civil disobedience, where activists plan to get arrested and know they will be prosecuted.

10. With respect to Clinton's election, some ACT UP members commented that many AIDS activists (in ACT UP and other organizations) naively believed that Clinton would provide more national leadership in fighting the AIDS crisis and that there would be less need to "act up."

11. Some activists learned about this history in ACT UP. Carrie, a white lesbian, stated: "Leftists in ACT UP/Chicago brought the lessons of COINTELPRO to AIDS activism. ACT UP was where I received my education about state repression, about the Black Panther Party, the Black Liberation Army, the Weather Underground, AIM, the Puerto Rican Independence Movement here in Chicago."

12. Government repression has been increasingly perpetrated recently within the context of the FBI's racist and xenophobic detainment of over 1,000 Muslims and people of Arab and South Asian descent in the aftermath of the September 11, 2001, terrorist attacks in New York City, Washington, D.C., and Pennsylvania. The *Los Angeles Times* (November 16, 2001) reported that no connection could be found between virtually any of these detainees and "terrorist groups." Furthermore, hundreds of immigrants from diverse national backgrounds have been detained, with no charges, under inhumane conditions by the INS for months (Nguyen 2002).

13. My analysis of the Denver case is based on newspaper articles, ACT UP/Chicago Legal Defense Committee literature, interviews with two defense committee members, and my own participation as a member of the Legal Defense Committee.

14. The Catholic Church has been the target of many ACT UP protests (see Arno and Feiden 1992; Carter 1992). ACT UP/Chicago's Legal Defense Committee literature described the goal of the ACT UP/Denver action: "Their message painted a picture of what a cemetery will look like in the not too distant future if the Catholic Church continues to oppose the use of condoms to prevent the spread of HIV: a cemetery in which tombstones relay AIDS as the cause of death."

15. On May 6, 1994, the three activists pled guilty to one deferred felony (which is expunged from criminal records after two years, barring

further convictions) and one misdemeanor. They were placed on probation. In addition, they were ordered to pay a fine of $2,900, perform community service, and write a letter of apology to the Catholic Church.

16. Unfortunately, more effective antiviral drugs, such as protease inhibitors, were not widely available until after most ACT UP chapters dissolved.

17. Social movement anthologies such as those edited by McAdam and Snow (1997) and Morris and Mueller (1992) contain little discussion of repression. The one chapter in Buechler and Cylke's (1997) anthology, by Marx (1997), ignores police brutality as well as the murder of prominent Black Panther Party, American Indian Movement, and Puerto Rican independence movement members—significant events during the period of the research.

18. Although none of the respondents spoke about gender in arrest situations or in cases of criminal prosecution, the harassment of women in ACT UP—presumably by the FBI—indicates that more research is needed to explore the relationship between gender and political repression.

19. According to Oberschall, "The means used will depend not just on constraints that other powerful groups impose upon the government, but on the characteristics of the subordinate classes and protesters as well" (Oberschall 1973: 256).

Chapter 6

1. More research is needed that focuses on outcomes as they relate to organizational ideology. How do outcomes differ in groups with a more inclusive consciousness versus a less inclusive consciousness?

References

Abu Jamal, Mumia. 1995. *Live from Death Row.* Reading, Mass.: Addison Wesley.

ACT UP/Chicago (AIDS Coalition to Unleash Power, Chicago). 1994. Prison Issues Committee documents.

ACT UP/New York (Aids Coalition to Unleash Power, New York) Women and AIDS Book Group. 1992. *Women, AIDS, and Activism.* Boston: South End Press.

Adam, Barry D. 1987. *The Rise of A Gay and Lesbian Movement.* Boston: Twayne Publishers.

———. 1989. "The AIDS Crisis." In *Feminist Frontiers,* ed. Laurel Richardson and Verta Taylor. Vol. 2. New York: Random House, pp. 306–309.

Allen, Robert. 1992. *Black Awakening in Capitalist America.* Trenton: Africa World Press.

Ames, Lynda J., Alana B. Atchinson, and D. Thomas Rose. 1994. "Community Building and Politics Among Gay Men: Empowerment Through AIDS?" Paper presented at the annual meeting of the American Sociological Association, Los Angeles, August.

Anastos, Kathryn, and Carola Marte. 1991. "Women: The Missing Persons in the AIDS Epidemic." In *The AIDS Reader: Social, Political, Ethical Issues,* ed. Nancy McKenzie. New York: Penguin Books.

Anzaldúa, Gloria. 1987. *Borderlands/La Frontera: The New Mestiza.* San Francisco: Aunt Lute Books.

———, ed. 1990. *Making Face, Making Soul—Haciendo Cara: Creative and Critical Perspectives by Feminists of Color.* San Francisco: Aunt Lute Books.

Anzaldúa, Gloria, and Cherríe Moraga, eds. 1983. *This Bridge Called My*

Back: Writings by Radical Women of Color. New York: Kitchen Table Women of Color Press.

Arno, Peter S., and Karyn L. Feiden, eds. 1992. *Against the Odds: The Story of AIDS Drug Development, Politics, and Profits.* New York: HarperCollins.

Baldwin, James. 1961. *Nobody Knows My Name.* New York: Dell Publishing.

———. 1972. *No Name in the Street.* New York: Dell Publishing.

Banzhaf, Marion. 1992. "Race, Women and AIDS." In *Women, AIDS and Activism* by the ACT UP/New York Women and AIDS Book Group. Boston: South End Press.

Beam, Joseph, ed. 1986. *In the Life: A Black Gay Anthology.* Boston: Alyson Publications.

Bennett, Lerone, Jr. 1984. *Before the Mayflower: A History of Black America.* New York: Penguin Books.

Braithwaite, Ronald L., and Ngina Lythcott. 1991. "Community Empowerment as a Strategy for Health Promotion for Black and Other Minority Populations." In *The AIDS Reader: Social, Political, Ethical Issues,* ed. Nancy F. McKenzie. New York: Penguin Books.

Bridges, George S., and Robert D. Crutchfield. 1988. "Law, Social Standing, and Racial Disparities in Imprisonment." *Social Forces* 66 (March): 699–724.

Buechler, Steven M., and F. Kurt Cylke Jr. 1997. *Social Movements: Perspectives and Issues.* Mountain View, Calif.: Mayfield Publishing.

Bulkin, Elly, Minnie Bruce Pratt, and Barbara Smith. 1988. *Yours in Struggle: Three Feminists' Perspectives on Anti-Semitism and Racism.* Ithaca, N.Y.: Firebrand Books.

Cameron, Barbara. 1983. "Gee, You Don't Seem Like an Indian from the Reservation." In *This Bridge Called My Back: Writings By Radical Women of Color,* ed. Gloria Anzaldúa and Cherríe Moraga. New York: Kitchen Table Women of Color Press.

Carson, Clayborn. 1996. *In Struggle: SNCC and the Black Awakening of the 1960s.* Cambridge, Mass.: Harvard University Press.

Carter, George M. 1992. "ACT-UP, the AIDS War, and Activism." Westfield, N.J.: Open Magazine Pamphlet Series.

Centers for Disease Control and Prevention. 1993. *HIV/AIDS Surveillance Report.* Atlanta: Centers for Disease Control and Prevention, July.

———. 1998. *Trends in the HIV and AIDS Epidemic.* Atlanta: Centers for Disease Control and Prevention.

———. 2000a. *HIV/AIDS Among African Americans.* Atlanta: Centers for Disease Control and Prevention, September.

———. 2000b. *Young People at Risk: HIV/AIDS Among America's Youth.* Atlanta: Centers for Disease Control and Prevention, September.

———. 2001. *HIV/AIDS Surveillance Report.* Atlanta: Centers for Disease Control and Prevention, August 22.

Chomsky, Noam. 1988. *Manufacturing Consent: The Political Economy of the Mass Media.* New York: Pantheon Books.

Christensen, K. 1992. "Prison Issues and HIV: Introduction." In *Women, AIDS and Activism* by the ACT UP/New York Women and AIDS Book Group. Boston: South End Press, pp. 139–142.

Churchill, Ward, and Jim Vander Wall. 1990. *Agents of Repression: The*

FBI's Secret Wars Against the Black Panther Party and the American Indian Movement. Boston: South End Press.

Clarke, Cheryl. 1983. "Lesbianism: An Act of Resistance." In *This Bridge Called My Back: Writings by Radical Women of Color,* ed. Gloria Anzaldúa and Cherríe Moraga. New York: Kitchen Table Women of Color Press.

Cohen, Cathy J. 1999. *The Boundaries of Blackness: AIDS and the Breakdown of Black Politics.* Chicago: University of Chicago Press.

Cohen, Jean. 1985. "Strategy or Identity: New Theoretical Paradigms and Contemporary Social Movements." *Social Research* 52: 663–716.

Cohen, Peter F. 1998. *Love and Anger: Essays on AIDS, Activism, and Politics.* Binghamton, N.Y.: Harrington Park Press.

Collins, Patricia Hill. 1990. *Black Feminist Thought: Knowledge, Consciousness, and the Politics of Empowerment.* Boston: Unwin Hyman.

———. 1993. "Toward a New Vision: Race, Class, and Gender as Categories of Analysis and Connection." *Race, Sex and Class* 1, no. 1 (Fall): 25–45.

Combahee River Collective. 1983. "The Combahee River Collective Statement." In *Home Girls: A Black Feminist Anthology,* ed. Barbara Smith. New York: Kitchen Table Women of Color Press.

Committee to End the Marion Lockdown. 1993. "The Nature of Imprisonment in the U.S. in Black and White." Chicago: Committee to End the Marion Lockdown, fall.

———. 1998. "Can't Jail the Spirit: Political Prisoners in the US." Chicago: Committee to End the Marion Lockdown.

Comstock, Gary. 1991. *Violence Against Lesbians and Gay Men.* New York: Columbia University Press.

Corea, Gena. 1992. *The Invisible Epidemic: The Story of Women and AIDS.* New York: HarperCollins.

Crimp, Douglas. 1990. *AIDS DEMO GRAPHICS.* Seattle: Bay Press.

Cruickshank, Margaret. 1992. *The Gay and Lesbian Liberation Movement.* New York: Routledge.

Dalton, Harlon L. 1991. "AIDS in Blackface." In *The AIDS Reader: Social, Political, Ethical Issues,* ed. Nancy F. McKenzie. New York: Penguin Books.

Davis, Angela, and Other Political Prisoners. 1971. *If They Come in the Morning.* New York: Joseph Okpaku Company.

———. 1983. *Women, Race, and Class.* New York: Vintage Books.

———. 1990. *Women, Culture, and Politics.* New York: Vintage Books.

Deitcher, David. 1995. *The Question of Equality: Lesbian and Gay Politics in America Since Stonewall.* New York: Scribner.

D'Emilio, John. 1983. *Sexual Politics, Sexual Communities: The Making of a Homosexual Minority in the United States, 1940–1970.* Chicago: University of Chicago Press.

Deresiewicz, William. 1991. "Against All Odds: Grass-roots Minority Groups Fight AIDS." In *The AIDS Reader: Social, Political, Ethical Issues,* ed. Nancy McKenzie. New York: Penguin Books.

Duberman, Martin. 1994. *Stonewall.* New York: Penguin Books.

Dunne, Bill. 1989. "The U.S. Penitentiary at Marion Illinois: An Instrument of Oppression." *New Studies on the Left* 14, nos. 1–2: 9–19.

Echols, Alice. 1989. *Daring to Be Bad: Radical Feminism in America, 1967–1975.* Minneapolis: University of Minnesota Press.

Elbaz, Gilbert. 1992. *The Sociology of AIDS Activism: The Case of ACT UP/ New York, 1987–1992*. Ph.D. diss., Department of Sociology, City University of New York.

Epstein, Steven. 1996. *Impure Science: AIDS, Activism, and the Politics of Knowledge*. Berkeley: University of California Press.

Fantasia, Rick. 1989. *Cultures of Solidarity: Consciousness, Action, and Contemporary American Workers*. Berkeley: University of California Press.

Farmer, Paul. 1996. "Women, Poverty, and AIDS." In *Women, Poverty, and AIDS: Sex, Drugs, and Structural Violence*, ed. Paul Farmer, Margaret Connors, and Janie Simmons. Boston: Common Courage Press.

Freedman, Estelle B., and John D'Emilio. 1988. *Intimate Matters: A History of Sexuality in America*. New York: Harper and Row.

Freeman, Jo. 1973. "The Origins of the Women's Liberation Movement." *American Journal of Sociology* 78, no. 4: 792–811.

Friedman, Debra, and Doug McAdam. 1992. "Collective Identity and Activism: Networks, Choices, and the Life of a Social Movement." In *Frontiers in Social Movement Theory*, ed. Aldon Morris and Carol Mueller. New Haven: Yale University Press.

Fullilove, Robert. 1995. "Community Disintegration and Public Health: A Case Study of New York City." In *Assessing the Social and Behavioral Science Base for HIV/AIDS Prevention and Intervention Workshop Summary*. Washington, D.C.: National Academy Press, pp. 93–116.

Gamson, Josh. 1989. "Silence, Death, and the Invisible Enemy: AIDS Activism and Social Movement 'Newness.'" *Social Problems* 36, no. 4 (October): 351–367.

Gamson, William A. 1989. *The Strategy of Social Protest*. Belmont, Calif.: Wadsworth.

———. 1992. "The Social Psychology of Collective Action," In *Frontiers in Social Movement Theory*, ed. Aldon Morris and Carol Mueller. New Haven: Yale University Press.

Giddings, Paula. 1984. *When and Where I Enter: The Impact of Black Women on Race and Sex in America*. New York: William Morrow.

Glick, Brian. 1989. *War at Home: Covert Action Against U.S. Activists and What We Can Do About It*. Boston: South End Press.

Goffman, Erving. 1961. *Asylums: Essays on the Social Situation of Mental Patients and Other Inmates*. Garden City, N.Y.: Doubleday.

Gould, Deborah Bejosa. 2000. *Sex, Death, and the Politics of Anger: Emotions and Reason in ACT UP's Fight Against AIDS*. Ph.D. diss., Department of Political Science, University of Chicago.

Gramsci, Antonio. 1987. *Prison Notebooks*. New York: International Publishers.

Gray, Jerry. 1991. "Panel Says Courts Are 'Infested with Racism.'" *New York Times*, June 5, p. B1.

Habermas, Jurgen. 1981. "New Social Movements." *Telos* 49: 33–37.

Hall, Jacquelyn Dowd. 1983. "The Mind That Burns in Each Body: Women, Rape and Racial Violence." In *The Powers of Desire: The Politics of Sexuality*, eds. Ann Snitow, Christine Stansell, and Sharon Thompson. New York: Monthly Review Press.

Hammonds, Evelynn. 1992. "Missing Persons: African American Women,

AIDS and the History of Disease." *Radical America* 24, no. 2 (July).

Harris, Craig G. 1986. "Cut Off from Among Their People." *In the Life,* ed. Joseph Beam. Boston: Alyson Publications.

Helmrich, William B. 1973. *The Black Crusaders: A Case Study of a Black Militant Organization.* New York: Harper and Row.

Hemphill, Essex, ed. 1991. *Brother to Brother: New Writings by Black Gay Men.* Boston: Alyson Publications.

Holman, Barry. 2001. *Masking the Divide: How Officially Reported Prison Statistics Distort the Racial and Ethnic Realities of Prison Growth.* Alexandria, Vir.: National Center on Institutions and Alternatives Research and Public Policy Report, May.

Jackson, George. 1970. *Soledad Brother: The Prison Letters of George Jackson.* New York: Bartam Books.

Julien, Isaac, and Kobena Mercer. 1991. "True Confessions: A Discourse on Images of Black Male Sexuality." In *Brother to Brother: New Writings by Black Gay Men,* ed. Essex Hemphill. Boston: Alyson Publications.

Kaye-Kantrowitz, Melanie. 1989. "Some Notes on Jewish Lesbian Identity." In *Nice Jewish Girls: A Lesbian Anthology,* ed. Evelyn Torton Beck. Boston: Beacon Press.

Kennedy, Elizabeth Lapovsky, and Madeline D. Davis. 1994. *Boots of Leather, Slippers of Gold: The History of a Lesbian Community.* New York: Penguin Books.

Killian, Lewis M. 1975. *The Impossible Revolution, Phase II: Black Power and the American Dream.* New York: Random House.

King, Deborah K. 1988. "Multiple Jeopardy, Multiple Consciousness: The Context of a Black Feminist Ideology." *Signs* 14, no. 1 (Autumn): 42–72.

Klandermans, Bert. 1988. "The Formation and Mobilization of Consensus." In *From Structure to Action: Comparing Movement Participation Across Cultures,* ed. Bert Klandermans, Hanspeter Kriesi, and Sidney Tarrow. International Social Movement Research Series, vol. 1. Greenwich, Conn.: JAI Press.

———. 1992. "The Social Construction of Protest and Multi-organizational Fields." In *The Frontiers in Social Movement Theory,* ed. Aldon Morris and Carol Mueller. New Haven, Conn.: Yale University Press.

Koopmans, Ruud. 1993. "The Dynamics of Protest Waves: West Germany, 1965–1989." *American Sociological Review* 58, no. 5 (October): 637–658.

Lengermann, Patricia Madoo, and Ruth A. Wallace. 1985. *Gender in America: Social Control and Social Change.* Englewood Cliffs, N.J.: Prentice-Hall.

Levenson, Jacob. 2000. "A Time for Healing." *Mother Jones,* July–August, pp. 42–47.

Lichenstein, Bronwen. 2001. "The AIDS Epidemic and Sociology Enquiry." *Footnotes* 29, no. 4 (April): 9.

Lipsky, Michael. 1968. "Protest as Political Resource." *American Political Science Review* 62: 1114–1158.

Lo, Clarence. 1992. "Communities of Challengers in Social Movement Theory." In *The Frontiers of Social Movement Frontier,* ed. Aldon Morris and Carol Mueller. New Haven, Conn.: Yale University Press.

Lorber, Judith. 2001. "Multiracial Feminism." In *Gender Mosaics,* ed. Dana

Vannoy. Los Angeles: Roxbury Publishing.

Lorde, Audre. 1982. *Zami: A New Spelling of My Name.* Freedom, Calif.: Crossing Press.

———. 1984. *Sister Outsider: Essays and Speeches.* Freedom, Calif.: Crossing Press.

Lusane, Clarence. 1991. *Pipe Dream Blues: Racism and the War on Drugs.* Boston: South End Press.

Mannheim, Karl. 1936. *Ideology and Utopia.* New York: Harcourt, Brace Jovanovich.

Marable, Manning. 1983. *How Capitalism Underdeveloped Black America: Problems in Race, Political Economy, and Society.* Boston: South End Press.

———. 1991. *Race, Reform, and Rebellion: The Second Reconstruction in Black America, 1945–1990.* Jackson: University Press of Mississippi.

Marx, Gary. 1974. "Thoughts on a Neglected Category of Social Movement Participant: The Agent Provocateur and the Informant." *American Journal of Sociology* 80: 402–442.

———. 1997. "External Efforts to Damage or Facilitate Social Movements: Some Patterns, Explanations, Outcomes, and Complications." In *Social Movements: Perspectives and Issues,* ed. Steven M. Buechler and F. Kurt Cylke Jr. Mountain View, Calif.: Mayfield Publishing.

Marx, Karl. 1977. *Capital.* Vol. 1. New York: Random House.

Mauer, Marc. 1990. *Young Black Men and the Criminal Justice System: A Growing National Problem.* Washington, D.C.: Sentencing Project, February.

McAdam, Doug. 1982. *Political Process and the Development of Black Insurgency, 1930–1970.* Chicago: University of Chicago Press.

———. 1983. "Tactical Innovation and the Pace of Insurgency." *American Sociological Review* 48: 735–754.

———. 1988. *Freedom Summer.* New York: Oxford University Press.

McAdam, Doug, John McCarthy, and Mayer Zald. 1988. "Social Movements." In *Handbook of Sociology,* ed. Neil Smelser. Newbury Park, Calif.: Sage.

McAdam, Doug, and David A. Snow. 1997. *Social Movements: Readings on Their Emergence, Mobilization, and Dynamics.* Los Angeles: Roxbury Publishing.

McCarthy, John D., and Mayer N. Zald. 1973. "The Trend in Social Movements in America: Professionalization and Resource Mobilization." Morristown, N.J.: General Learning Press.

McKenzie, Nancy F., ed. 1991. *The AIDS Reader: Social, Political, Ethical Issues.* New York: Penguin Books.

Melucci, Alberto. 1989. *Nomads of the Present: Social Movements and Individual Needs in Contemporary Society.* London: Hutchinson Radius.

Miller, Heather G., Charles F. Turner, and Lincoln E. Moses, eds. 1990. *AIDS: The Second Decade* (Summary). Washington, D.C.: National Resource Council, National Academy Press.

Morris, Aldon D. 1984. *The Origins of the Civil Rights Movement: Black Communities Organizing for Change.* New York: Macmillan.

———. 1992. "Political Consciousness and Collective Action." In *The Frontiers of Social Movement Theory,* ed. Aldon Morris and Carol Mueller. New Haven, Conn.: Yale University Press.

————. 1993. "Birmingham Confrontation Reconsidered: An Analysis of the Dynamics and Tactics of Mobilization." *American Sociological Review* 58, no. 5 (October).

Morris, Aldon, and Cedric Herring. 1987. "Theory and Research in Social Movements: A Critical Review." *Annual Review of Political Science,* ed. Samuel Long. Vol. 2. Norwood, N.J.: Ablex Publishing, pp. 139–198.

Morris, Aldon, and Carol McClurg Mueller. 1992. *The Frontiers of Social Movement Theory.* New Haven, Conn.: Yale Univeristy Press.

Mueller, Carol McClurg. 1992. "Building Social Movement Theory." In *The Frontiers of Social Movement Theory,* ed. Aldon Morris and Carol Mueller. New Haven, Conn.: Yale University Press.

National Center on Institutions and Alternatives. 1992. "Hobbling a Generation: Young African American Males in the Criminal Justice System of America's Cities: Baltimore, Maryland." News Release. National Center on Institutions and Alternatives, Alexandria, Va., September 1, 1992.

Navarro, Raymond. 1991. "AIDS Activist Prodded Chicano Community." *The Guardian,* November 28.

Nguyen, Tram. 2002. "Detained or Disappeared?" *ColorLines Magazine* 5, no. 2 (Summer), pp. 4–7.

Oberschall, Anthony. 1973. *Social Conflict and Social Movements.* Englewood Cliffs, N.J.: Prentice Hall.

————. 1978. "The Decline of the 1960s Social Movements." In *Research in Social Movements, Conflict, and Change,* Volume 1, ed. Louis Kriesberg. Greenwich, Conn.: JAI, pp. 257–289.

Oegema, Dirk, and Bert Klandermans. 1994. "Why Social Movement Sympathizers Don't Participate." *American Sociological Review* 59, no. 5 (October).

O'Melveny, Mary. 1989. "U.S. Political Prison: Lexington Prison High Security Unit." *New Studies on the Left* 14, nos. 1–2: 37–43.

Opp, Karl-Dieter, and Christiane Gern. 1993. "Dissident Groups, Personal Networks, and Spontaneous Cooperation: The East German Revolution of 1989." *American Sociological Review* 58, no. 5 (October).

O'Reilly, Kenneth. 1989. *Racial Matters: The FBI's Secret File on Black America, 1960–1972.* New York: Macmillan.

Padgug, Robert A. 1989. "Gay Villain, Gay Hero: Homosexuality and the Social Construction of AIDS." In *Passion and Power: Sexuality in History,* ed. Kathy Peiss and Christina Simmons, with Robert Padgug. Philadelphia: Temple University Press.

Parenti, Michael. 1988. *Democracy for the Few.* New York: St. Martin's Press.

Patton, Cindy. 1990. *Inventing AIDS.* New York: Routledge.

Payne, Charles M. 1996. *I've Got the Light of Freedom: The Organizing Tradition and the Mississippi Freedom Struggle.* Berkeley: University of California Press.

Perez, Emma. 1991. "Sexuality and Discourse: Notes From a Chicana Survivor." In *Chicana Lesbians: The Girls Our Mothers Warned Us About,* ed. Carla Trujillo. Berkeley, Calif.: Third Woman Press.

Peters, Howard, Director, Illinois Department of Corrections. 1993. Letter to Debbie Gould, ACT UP/Chicago, June 18.

Piven, Frances Fox, and Richard A. Cloward. 1977. *Poor People's Movements: Why They Succeed, How They Fail.* New York: Vintage Books.

PWA RAG (Prisoners with AIDS Rights Advocacy Group). 1993. *Quarterly Newsline* 6, no. 5.

Reiman, Jeffrey. 1995. *The Rich Get Richer and the Poor Get Prison: Ideology, Crime, and Criminal Justice.* Needham Heights, Mass.: Allyn and Bacon.

Rich, Adrienne. 1986. *Blood, Bread, and Poetry: Selected Prose, 1979–1985.* New York: W. W. Norton.

Riggs, Marlon. 1989. *Tongues Untied* (film). Signifyin' Works.

Roscigno, Vincent J. 1994. "Social Movement Struggle and Race, Gender, and Class Inequality." *Race, Sex and Class* 2, no. 1 (Fall): 109–126.

Rothenberg, Paula S. 2002. *White Privilege: Essential Readings on the Other Side of Racism.* New York: Worth Publishers.

Saalfield, Catherine. 1992. "Intravenous Drug Use, Women and HIV." In *Women, AIDS, and Activism* by the ACT UP/New York Women and AIDS Book Group. Boston: South End Press.

Schneider, Beth E. 1992. "AIDS and Class, Race, and Gender Relations." In *The Social Context of AIDS,* ed. Joan Huber and Beth Schneider. Newbury Park, Calif.: Sage.

Schoepf, Brooke, Claude Schoepf, and Joyce V. Millen. 2000. "Theoretical Therapies, Remote Remedies: SAPs and the Political Ecology of Poverty and Health in Africa." In *Dying for Growth: Global Inequality and the Health of the Poor,* ed. Jim Yong Kim, Joyce V. Millen, Alec Irwin, and John Gersham. Monroe, Me.: Common Courage Press.

Scott, James. 1985. Weapons of the Weak. New Haven: Yale University Press.

Sellers, Cleveland. 1973. *The River of No Return: The Autobiography of a Black Militant and the Life and Death of SNCC.* New York: William Morrow.

Shakur, Assata. 1987. *Assata: An Autobiography.* Chicago: Lawrence Hill Books.

Shilts, Randy. 1987. *And the Band Played On.* New York: St. Martin's Press.

Slade, E., and M. Sweney. 1992. *Acting Up for Prisoners* (video). ACT UP/San Francisco.

Smith, Barbara. 1993. "Homophobia: Why Bring It Up?" In *The Lesbian and Gay Studies Reader,* ed. Henry Abelove, Michele Aina Barale, and David M. Halperin. New York: Routledge.

———, ed. 1983. *Home Girls: A Black Feminist Anthology.* New York: Kitchen Table: Women of Color Press.

Snow, David, and Robert Benford. 1988. "Ideology, Frame Resonance, and Participant Mobilization." In *From Structure to Action: Comparing Social Movement Research Across Cultures,* ed. Bert Klandermans, Hanspeter Kriesi, and Sidney Tarrow. International Social Movement Research Series, vol. 1. Greenwich, Conn.: JAI Press.

Snow, David A., E. Burke Rochford, Steven K. Worden, and Robert D. Benford. 1986. "Frame Alignment Processes, Micromobilization, and Movement Participation." *American Sociological Review* 51, no. 4 (August): 464–481.

"Special Section on the Prison Industrial Complex." 1998. *ColorLines Magazine* 1, no. 2 (Fall).

Spector, Malcolm, and John I. Kitsuse. 1987. *Constructing Social Problems.* New York: Aldine De Gruyter.

Stockdill, Brett. 1995. "(Mis)Treating Prisoners with AIDS: Analyzing Health Care Behind Bars." In *The Sociology of Health Care*, ed. Jennie Jacobs Kronenfeld. Vol. 12. Greenwich, Conn.: JAI Press.

———. 2000. "ACT UP." In *Encyclopedia of Gay History,* ed. by George Haggerty. New York: Garland Press.

———. 2001a. "Forging a Multidimensional Oppositional Consciousness: Lessons from Community Based AIDS Activism." *Oppositional Consciousness: The Subjective Roots of Social Protest,* ed. Jane Mansbridge and Aldon Morris. Chicago: University of Chicago Press.

———. 2001b. "Blood at the Roots: A Structural Analysis of Racist Violence." *Journal of Social and Behavioral Sciences* 38, no. 2 (Spring): 139–160.

Stolen Lives: Killed by Law Enforcement. 1999. The Stolen Lives Project. New York: Anthony Baez Foundation; October 22nd Coalition to Stop Police Brutality. Los Angeles: National Lawyers Guild.

Stoller, Nancy E. 1998. *Lessons from the Damned: Queers, Whores, and Junkies Respond to AIDS.* New York: Routledge.

Tagle, Richard. 1993. *Assessing the HIV-Prevention Needs of Gay and Bisexual Men of Color.* U.S. Conference of Mayors and the U.S. Conference of Local Health Officers

Tarrow, Sidney. 1992. "Mentalities, Political Cultures, and Collective Action Frames: Constructing Meanings Through Action." In *Frontiers of Social Movement Theory,* ed. Aldon Morris and Carol Mueller. New Haven, Conn.: Yale University Press.

Taylor, Verta. 1989. "The Future of Feminism: A Social Movement Analysis." In *Feminist Frontiers II,* ed. Laurel Richardson and Verta Taylor. New York: Random House.

Taylor, Verta, and Nancy Whittier. 1992. "Collective Identity in Social Movement Communities: Lesbian Feminist Mobilization." In *Frontiers of Social Movement Theory,* ed. Aldon Morris and Carol Mueller. New Haven, Conn.: Yale University Press.

Tilly, Charles. 1978. *From Mobilization to Revolution.* Reading, Mass.: Addison-Wesley.

Trujillo, Carla, ed. 1991. *Chicana Lesbians: The Girls Our Mothers Warned Us About.* Berkeley, Calif.: Third Woman Press.

Uekert, Brenda K. 1994. "State Terrorism and Armed Conflict: Is Terrorism an Effective Strategy?" Paper presented at the Annual Meeting of the American Sociological Association, Los Angeles.

U.S. Bureau of the Census. 2001. *United States Census 2000.* Washington, D.C.: U.S. Census Bureau. March.

U.S. Department of Justice, Office of Justice Programs, Bureau of Justice Statistics. 1991. *Survey of State Prison Inmates, 1991.* Washington, D.C.: U.S. Department of Justice, p. 3.

———. 2001. "Bulletin: Prison and Jail Inmates at Midyear 2000." Washington, D.C.: U.S. Department of Justice, March.

"Voices: Women of ACE (AIDS Counseling and Education), Bedford Hills Correctional Facility." 1992. In *Women, AIDS and Activism* by the ACT UP/New York Women and AIDS Book Group. Boston: South End Press, pp. 143–155.

Walker, Jackie. 1992. "Condom Distribution." *The National Prison Project*

Journal 7, no. 4: 26.

Weeks, Jeffrey. 1992. *Against Nature: Essays on History, Sexuality and Identity.* London: River Orams Press.

White, Robert W., and Terry Falkenberg White. 1994. "Repression and the Liberal State: The Case of Northern Ireland, 1969–1972." Paper presented at the Annual Meeting of the American Sociological Association in Los Angeles.

Whitman, S. 1991. *The Crime of Black Imprisonment.* Chicago: Committee to End the Marion Lockdown.

Wolfe, Laura. 1993. "Denver Grand Jury." Unpublished manuscript.

Women in the Director's Chair. 1994. *(Mis)Treating Prisoners with AIDS* (video). Chicago: Women in the Director's Chair and ACT UP/Chicago.

Zald, Mayer. 1992. "Looking Backward to Look Forward: Reflections on the Past and Future of the Resource Mobilization Program." In *The Frontiers of Social Movement Theory,* ed. Aldon Morris and Carol Mueller. New Haven, Conn.: Yale University Press.

Zimbardo, Philip. 1985. "The Pathology of Imprisonment." In *Down to Earth Sociology,* ed. J. M. Henslin. New York: Macmillan.

Zinn, Maxine Baca, and Bonnie Thorne Dill. 1997. "Theorizing Difference from Multiracial Feminism." In *Through the Prism of Difference: Readings on Sex and Gender,* ed. Maxine Baca Zinn, Pierrette Hondagneu-Sotelo, and Michael A. Messner. Needham Heights, Mass.: Allyn and Bacon.

Index

ACT UP (AIDS Coalition to Unleash Power): classism and, 44; and communities of color, 66–67; criminal prosecution of, 140–142; decline of, 109, 114, 135; direct action tactics of, 6, 93, 107–110; divergent framings of AIDS in, 149–150; FBI surveillance of, 139–140; formation and goal of, 6; and health care system demonstrations, 136–137; importance of, 164; inclusivity and radical change efforts in, 145–146; internal education campaigns of, 59; and LGBT mainstream community, 117; membership of, 6; militant politic of, 156; partial oppositional consciousness in, 84; people of color caucuses in, 40; police brutality toward, 136–139, 145; political divisions in, 90–91; political repression of, 117, 135–143; prison activism of, 3; racism and, 40–41, 76; radical lesbians' role in, 117–118; singular crisis perspective in, 32, 34; sexism in, 37–38; and threat of brutality, 145; women's caucuses in, 91, 158

ACT UP/Chicago, 32; confrontational tactics of, 59–60; disintegration of, 109, 114

ACT UP/Chicago's Prison Issues Committee, 21, 83, 92–120, 140; "agitprop" tactic of, 102; and antiprisoner sentiment, 100, 113; consciousness raising campaigns of, 103–107; direct action tactics of, 107–112; emergence of, 91; frame alignment strategies of, 101–106; lack of political support for, 112–113; media coverage of, 108, 110, 111; members of, 92–95; and organizing in communities of color, 113–114; and prisoner empowerment, 98–99, 119; strategies of, 96–110; successes of, 114–115; and tactical interactions/innovations, 111–112; and third-party debate, 115–119

About the Book

AIDS has claimed the lives of nearly 500,000 people in the United States and has become the focus of intense political activism. Brett Stockdill reveals that people living with HIV/AIDS are often multiply oppressed—gay men of color, for example—and explores how interlocking oppressions fragment activism and thus impede AIDS prevention and intervention. Demonstrating that a unified approach to issues of race, class, gender, and sexuality can most effectively combat the AIDS epidemic, he highlights critical links among sociological analysis, public policy, and activism.

Brett C. Stockdill is an assistant professor of sociology at California State Polytechnic University at Pomona.